*Carlton Fredericks'*
New *Low Blood Sugar*
*and You*

# Carlton Fredericks' New *Low Blood Sugar* and You

Carlton Fredericks, PhD

A Perigee Book

Perigee Books
are published by
The Berkley Publishing Group
200 Madison Avenue
New York, New York 10016

The author gratefully acknowledges permission from The Bobbs-Merrill Company, Inc.,
to quote from *The Food Connection,* copyright © 1979 by David Sheinkin, M.D.,
Michael Schachter, M.D., and Richard Hutton.

The author wishes to thank Ruth Sperling for making the graphs
of the blood sugar curves.

Book design by Constance Sohodski

Library of Congress Cataloging in Publication Data

Fredericks, Carlton.
Carlton Fredericks' *new* low blood sugar and you.

Includes index.
1. Hypoglycemia.   2. Hypoglycemia—Diet therapy—
Recipes.   I. Title.
RC662.F73   1984      616.4′66      84-7066
ISBN 0-399-51087-7 (pbk.)

Cover design © 1985 by One Plus One Studio

First Perigee printing, 1985
Printed in the United States of America

30   29   28   27

It was the early 1920's. Physicians were becoming somewhat disillusioned with the new "answer to diabetes," for it seemed impossible to predict when a dose of insulin would drop the blood sugar dangerously low, subjecting the diabetic to insulin shock and all its profound impacts on body and mind.

While the profession was groping to protect its diabetic patients from this unanticipated danger, a medical pioneer realized that he was viewing identical signs in nondiabetics who were *not* being treated with insulin. In 1924, he published his observations in a major medical journal, tracing many bizarre mental and physical signs and symptoms to chronic low blood sugar caused by an excess of internally produced insulin.

In an instance of true medical serendipity, he indicted the surfeit of sugar and caffeine in the American diet as a prime cause of this type of pancreatic overactivity and consequent chronic low blood sugar. He cannot be faulted for the disappearance of his paper in the cultural lag, with the result that victims of low blood sugar have been mistakenly labeled neurotics, psychotics, psychasthenics, hysterics, "constitutionally inadequates," or malingerers.

To those who have needlessly suffered and to that medical pioneer, Dr. Seale Harris, I dedicate this book.

*Carlton Fredericks, PhD*

And to Rose, who gave me her precious daughter and made me a beloved son. I miss her.

C.F.

# Contents

# *Preface*

This book was written for you if you suffer from or would like to avoid:

Anxiety attacks, unpredictable and apparently out of the blue
Panic attacks, similarly unjustified by your life situation
Depression, also for no apparent reason
Epilepsy
Schizophrenia
Agoraphobia
Claustrophobia
Tinnitus (noises in your ears)
Obesity, with an uncontrollable addiction for sweets
Obsessive-compulsive behavior
Allergies, particularly multiple
Difficulties with short-term memory and concentration
Repeated vaginal yeast infections
Depersonalized feelings

When you discover in reading this text that the common denominator frequently behind such symptoms is your diet, and that the remedy is a change in your eating habits, your reaction is likely to be: "If this is true, how is it my doctor never mentioned it to me?"

There is a fundamental problem in the practice of medicine, perhaps best described by Montaigne long ago. He said that when a medical innovation is first discovered, it's not true. Twenty years later, it's true, but it's not important. After another twenty years, it's true, it's important, but it isn't new, and we have something better now anyway. That describes the lag for which medicine is notorious. There are some classic examples of the delay in accepting new findings and innovative thinking. Consider, for instance, that papers on the Pap smear were published for ten years before the researcher could capture the attention of his fellow physicians. Remember that Fleming was considered a little odd for his belief that molds produce an antibiotic that can be used in the treatment of human infections. (It's called penicillin now.) Remember that the first electrocardiogram was not only rejected by the American Medical Association, but was called "electronic quackery." It should not be astonishing, then, that this same medical association has taken exactly the same attitude toward the nutritional therapies described in this and many other books. Moreover, that attitude has been very ambivalent. Initially, the association awarded a gold medal to Dr. Seale Harris, the pioneer in recognizing that sugar is a mischief maker for many patients. Thirty years later, the AMA announced that such criticisms of sugar are made by medical charlatans preying upon the gullible public. Only five years after that, the same medical association gave a course for physicians, to teach them how to recognize the mischief created by excessive sugar intake in those sensitive to it.

The lag becomes even more of a trap for a suffering public when the psychiatrists enter the arena. An old friend, Dr. Emanuel Cheraskin, who is a physician and a dentist, as well as a medical nutritionist, has been heard to remark that if it were possible to remove your head and mail it to a psychiatrist, he would probably treat it. The remark simply emphasizes the failure of psychiatrists to remember that they are physicians, that the mind-body relationship is a two-way road, and that there are physical disorders which can cause symptoms that appear to be purely emotional. This is not a light matter. Some years ago, 115 patients who were being treated by psychiatrists for "emotional" problems were carefully examined by a team of competent physicians, which found all 115 to be suffering from physical disorders that were responsible for their symptoms (see page 18). I bring this up because a number of the disorders listed at the opening of this preface have been treated as if they were purely psychiatric problems. I have been known to jest that the psychoanalyst will tell you that your unjustified fears derive from the fact that your parents bought a square toilet seat, with the result that you have felt cornered ever since. The joke becomes pallid when you listen to a psychiatrist solemnly declare that fear of elevators derives from the fact that your father was not upwardly mobile. That kind of jargon has deprived many patients of needed physical examinations and required physical treatment.

Hence, this book. In its first edition, published in 1969, it was bought by close to a million Americans, and my files are filled with letters of gratitude from patients who, by simple changes in their dietary habits, escaped the psychiatric couch and the endless list of drugs. You will find some of those letters mentioned here in this text.

It is a source of pride for me that the wide distribution of *Low Blood Sugar and You* came in large part from recommendation or distribution of the book by physicians. Given the lack of nutrition courses in medical curricula, I anticipated that it would take decades before medical men came to recognize that we of the Western world are eating an abnormal diet, including, among other nutritional obscenities, a teaspoonful of sugar every thirty-five minutes, twenty-four hours a day. Following that, these physicians then had to proceed to the realization that the average American diet is a basis for physical and "emotional" disorders, which are not appropriately treated with drugs. From that reorientation of medical thinking, though, it was then but a short step in medical practice to institute correction of diet. Watching the responses in the disorders I have listed, physicians were irrevocably committed to a philosophy that Hippocrates voiced many centuries ago. In essence, he said: "Try diet first."

I must add a note of admiration for the practitioners who have had the courage to leave the mainstream of drug-oriented medicine, thereby subjecting themselves to the enormous pressures of the orthodox medical establishment. In thinking of them, I am often reminded of a remark made in a Nobel Prize acceptance speech, to the effect that it is a wise herd that does not too severely punish its deviants, for while they are idiots and criminals, they are also prophets and discoverers.

This text does not present panaceas. There is no one therapy that is effective for everybody with the same disorder, nor are the degrees of response the same in those who do respond. Neither does this text advise self-treatment. Indeed, in some instances that would be impossible, for preliminary testing is a very real requirement in some disorders.

The supervision of a medical nutritionist—and there is now a considerable body of them—is more often than not an excellent investment, and in Appendix I, I provide names of medical societies which emphasize nutrition, so that should you find it necessary, you can obtain referral to an expert.

In the sixteen years since *Low Blood Sugar and You* was written, I have become even more disillusioned about the glucose-tolerance test, which is the device most frequently used for diagnosing both diabetes and hypoglycemia. Examination of one drop of blood can establish the diagnosis of diabetes, but the conventional glucose-tolerance test for low blood sugar, properly given, requires administration of a concentrated sugary drink and repeated withdrawals of blood to study the dynamics of sugar metabolism, rather than the blood sugar level at a given moment. I am frequently persuaded that therapeutic diagnosis does just as well, given that diabetes is not present. This means placing the suspected hypoglycemic on the correct diet and watching his response. If, after a month or two, his symptoms are significantly reduced, the diagnosis has been established.

My objections to the glucose-tolerance test are based on the fact that it is administered in the peace and quiet of the laboratory or the physician's office. It thereby may not duplicate the dynamics of the patient's sugar metabolism when he is engaged in normal activities. To me, it would be more realistic and certainly more revealing to have the patient report early in the morning, for a fasting blood sugar determination, and then to follow that with breakfast, with sugar determinations a half hour and an hour later. At that point, the patient would go back to his normal activities, reporting for another sugar test before lunch, after lunch, and in midafternoon. From what I have observed in the practice of clinical nutrition, the results of such a "normal activities" test may frequently be quite different from those that accrue from the laboratory procedure. I am particularly anxious to avoid the glucose-tolerance test for children, for obvious reasons. Here I think therapeutic diagnosis is indispensable if one is not to inflict on youngsters the trauma of repeated withdrawals of blood.

Since this book was written, I have also learned that the conventional glucose-tolerance test, sampling the blood sugar level at half-hour, one-hour, two-hour, three-hour, four-hour, five-hour, and six-hour intervals, may miss significant changes in blood sugar levels. Very simply, there is no law which requires that drops or rises in blood sugar must occur on the hour. Close surveillance of the patient for any symptoms is indispensable, and when symptoms appear, levels of blood sugar should be tested. In this way, deviations that otherwise would never be detected may be determined and accurately measured.

Among my sources of dissatisfaction with the glucose-tolerance test is the fact that glucose is the test substance. Glucose is sugar, but a special type of sugar that is not ordinarily consumed by the public. The public eats sucrose. Sucrose, ordinary white sugar, is 50 percent glucose and 50 percent fructose. Fructose itself has been indicated as a trouble-maker for some people. Therefore, testing for glucose alone does not make too much scientific sense. It also introduces a variable, for glucose is made from corn, and in some exquisitely sensitive individuals, the reaction may be an allergy to corn, rather than a disturbance of glucose metabolism.

Low blood sugar frequently plays an important role in asthma and other allergies. Not only can allergic reactions cause a drop in blood sugar, but they can cause a sharp rise, indicating that investigation for allergy is indispensable in the management of diabetes, though it is seldom performed. Allergy is capable of causing all the symptoms of low blood sugar, with or without a drop in sugar level. When patients are definitely hypoglycemic but don't respond to or even worsen on the hypoglycemia diet, the possibility that the patient is allergic to some of the good foods recommended in that diet must be recognized.

Some patients' failure to respond to the hypoglycemia diet is based on the need for more or less carbohydrate than such diets ordinarily supply. As little as 20 grams of carbohydrate, up or down, may make the difference between the successfully treated patient and the one who does not respond.

In the pre-breakfast drink recommended with the menus in this book, I suggest the use of glycine (aminoacetic acid). This is the simplest of all amino (protein) acids—a harmless food supplement which has been very beneficial to hypoglycemics. For some years, the Food and Drug Administration labeled glycine as a food additive, which effectively took it off the market, despite protests that it is normal to the diet and the body and beneficial to the hypoglycemic, particularly in the hypoglycemia symptoms occurring in the "Morgagni syndrome." Glycine has now been restored to respectability, which is a relief, because the only substitute is whole gelatin. Whole gelatin is 27 percent glycine, but it may contain a significant amount of fluorides, for which malnourished people may have a poor tolerance.

In the past sixteen years I have had considerable experience with the use of glycerin as a supplement of the hypoglycemia diet. In the average person, glycerin is converted directly into glycogen (stored sugar), on which the person can draw as his body needs fuel in times of deprivation. Thus glycerin does not usually trigger a pancreatic reaction, as does sugar itself. It acts instead as a kind of "time capsule" or stored energy. A tablespoon in water between meals (or at other intervals, as specified by the physician) often dramatically "recharges the batteries," particularly for patients with the "flat curve" of glucose tolerance. Some individuals are allergic to glycerin, however, though it is a normal by-product of the metabolism of fats in the body.

Another device that is helpful for some hypoglycemics requires breakfast and then return to bed for an hour. In many cases, this lets them face the day's demands with a better capacity for work and stress.

In testing for hypoglycemia by the conventional glucose-tolerance method, I have observed that stress, applied at about the fourth hour of the procedure, may elicit the full-blown symptoms of low blood sugar in a patient who would otherwise react normally. The stress may be as minimal as a few minutes of running on a treadmill, a short period of hyperventilation (breathing in and out with abnormal rapidity), or breathing into and from a paper bag. In some patients who were observed closely, psychotic behavior has been provoked by the stress test, sometimes revealing that the patient was actually suffering from both a type of schizophrenia and hypoglycemia—not an infrequent combination. This, not at all incidentally, means that such patients can be helped by dietary control.

There are physicians who will assure you that hypoglycemia is extremely rare, or that it is an imaginary disease, seized upon by neurotics who are seeking a physical explanation for their symptoms and who are being exploited by venal and obviously incompetent physicians. If you encounter this from a medical practitioner, you might suggest that he write to the Carbohydrate Laboratory of the United States Department of Agriculture. Serenely indifferent to this type of medical propaganda, that laboratory conducted a test for the tolerance of sugar in the amounts eaten by average Americans. They found that so large a percentage of the subjects reacted abnormally that, as private citizens rather than employees of the Department of Agriculture, they wrote to the FDA suggesting that sugar should no longer be considered GRAS ("generally regarded as safe")—in other words, that the food industry should be required to prove that sugar in large quantities, as we eat it, is safe. As you read this book, you will be driven to agreement with them. That one decision may be your most important dietary contribution to your good health.

Carlton Fredericks, PhD
New City, New York
1984

# Introduction

As your doctor puts it, you've been through "all the tests," and the results are "essentially negative," which means he didn't find heart trouble, cancer, high blood pressure, gastric ulcer, hardening of the arteries, glaucoma, lupus erythematosus, or emphysema.

You are now one of the elite—you belong to the very small minority of healthy Americans, healthy with the exception of your sinus trouble, postnasal drip, colds, viruses, allergies, constipation, dandruff, poor circulation, fatigability, blotchy skin, sensitivity to sunshine, and falling hair. *Physically* you're fine. The emotional troubles, which brought you to the doctor in the first place, are still unexplained and unremedied: you're nervous, irritable, sleepless, tired, edgy, and subject to uncontrollable fits of temper, difficulties in concentrating, hypochondria, and a completely unjustified, constant feeling of "something terrible about to happen." You can't stand crowds, telephone booths, subways, elevators, shopping in busy supermarkets and department stores, or any additional doses of tranquilizers and sleeping pills. And you will go out of your mind if once again you hear that it's "all in your mind."

And this is obviously where your doctor is going to place it, because there's nothing else left to blame it all on. It's the reaction to your spouse's peculiarities; it's the guilt about that extramarital adventure, or the tension from lack of one; it's the monotony of the job or the housekeeping; it's your failure as a parent, or your failure to become one; it's *your* parents' failures as a pair of parents . . . and on and on it goes.

This procedure—the ruling out of physical disease, which leaves nothing but the emotional to blame—is called "diagnosis by exclusion." Only when physical disorders have been ruled out may the emotional be considered; and this becomes the most frequent pathway into psychotherapy or psychoanalysis. It isn't so bad if it turns out to be "all in your mind"; after all, the stigma of going to a psychiatrist has vanished. Even medical men go to psychiatrists now, and, as a result of this, a steadily increasing percentage of their diagnoses falls into the psychosomatic area. But there is one frequent and fatal flaw in the usual procedure of diagnosis by exclusion. The exclusion must be *total.* All possible physical disorders must be screened out. The spectrum of examinations and tests must be complete, and the doctor thereby sure that he has not missed *anything.*

But he does miss—and frequently, at that. He errs in many ways. When he does diagnose a physical illness, he may be far off target. Autopsy reports show a frightening difference between actual and supposed causes of death. Other diagnostic errors were revealed; for instance, in a re-study of 115 patients who were referred for psychological treatment on the basis of diagnosis by exclusion. All 115, on competent, careful reexamination, were found to have physical ailments that were actually the causes of their "emotional" symptoms. Correct diagnosis ultimately resulted in the cure of 45 and the improvement of 36 of these patients. Three did not respond. Tragically, 31 others died within a few years, 25 of them from *cancer.* Had they heeded the American Medical Association (AMA) advice to seek frequent checkups to prevent cancer? Two errors in the prior examinations of these people are obvious: patient histories were superficially taken; examinations could not have been competent and total.

There are other errors that place people on a psychiatric couch who should instead be in a hospital bed. A physician who is not looking for a specific disorder is not likely to find it. A high index of suspicion is needed if we are to have a low level of misses. A patient who withholds facts, symptoms, family history, or other relevant information may lead an unsuspicious physician astray. A doctor who allows fifteen minutes for a first interview—and there are many such, unfortunately—will tend to lean on the laboratory rather than on his diagnostic acumen, for which there is no substitute. Even in the selection of tests there is a bias that may introduce error or omission, for there are literally thou-

sands of tests that can be used to appraise a person's health or deviations from it. The doctor will obviously order *some* of these. Experience
and sound judgment will, hopefully, dictate his choices and his omis-
sions. If these factors are not operative, the wrong tests may be given,
the critical ones omitted.

There is also the factor of timing: the right test may be ordered at the
wrong moment. There is, as an example, an enzyme test for inflammation of the pancreas, which, administered when the patient is having
no pain, gives false assurance that all is well. Don't dismiss this as
academic. One woman, assured that her abdominal pain had to be
emotional in origin, went into three years of expensive psychoanalysis.
Tens of thousands of dollars later, with no relief from her suffering, she
underwent that same enzyme test again—at the right moment, which
was at the height of her pain. So it was that a relatively unknown
doctor found what the high-priced specialists had missed—pan-
creatitis—and by the stroke of a pen, the patient was converted from a
"severely neurotic" person to a victim of a very real and quite definitely
physical disease. The tale is mentioned with special emphasis; it forms
part of the motivation for writing this book, especially since the patient
was a member of the family of the author.

Medicine boasts of, rather than apologizes for, the development of
diagnosis by computer. But medicine is an art as well as an emerging
science, and computers can but confirm what has been suggested by the
diagnostic acumen of a competent physician with a high level of suspicion. Computer analysis should never establish a diagnosis; it should
merely confirm one. As long as medicine considers computers as peers,
rather than as aids, just as long will patients be referred to psychiatrists
on the basis of diagnosis by exclusion that has not excluded all.

Other sources of error reside in the laboratory. There are sometimes
critical differences in test results from two different technicians, both
competent, though robot chemists are fast eliminating these errors.
Laboratories nonetheless make mistakes, inadvertently, carelessly, or
criminally. So it is that the cautious physician will eliminate these
sources of error by sending identical samples to two different laboratories, or two samples to the same laboratory, the samples labeled as if
from two different patients.

It should be apparent by now that this book will deal with certain physical disorders that are capable of mimicking emotional disturbances and mental disease. These sicknesses can start with tension, with vitamin deficiency or an imbalanced diet, with a disturbance in body chemistry, with allergy, even with a virus infection. All the symptoms overlap, even though the causes are so different, for the brain and the nervous system have limited ways in which to express reaction to insult.

And all the symptoms argue for the label "psychosomatic," because they include depression, irritability, anxiety, fears, difficulties in concentration and with the memory span, unjustified weeping, insomnia, fatigue, inability to make decisions, sensitivity to slight noises, and ferocious temper tantrums. All or some of these complaints frequently may be complicated by sexual frigidity, nightmares, shortness of breath, dizziness, blurred vision, thoughts of suicide, panic, and anxiety attacks.

Look back over that list. If these are your complaints, and you so describe them to the average physician, will he not talk to you gently about your relationship to your spouse, job, employer, family, children, and early childhood? How long will it be before he reaches for his prescription pad to prescribe sedatives, sleeping drugs, or tranquilizers? How long before he suggests a psychiatrist? You can't blame him much because that list of symptoms is described in his textbooks as marking the patient as "typically neurotic." It's obviously all in your mind—except that, sometimes, it isn't. It may be a physical disease, of a type which can slip through his "complete physical checkup"—if, indeed, he gives you one.

There is a risk in telling you this. You may decide that all diagnoses of emotional and mental disorders are suspect, all psychological treatment unwarranted. Don't do what the medical profession itself did. It called Sigmund Freud a crackpot; it laughed Smith Jelliffe off the platform when that distinguished doctor, twenty years ahead of his time, proposed the concept of "psychosomatic" disorders. It was not until much later that medical men leaped aboard the psychosomatic bandwagon, to the point where today you must crawl into the physician's office on hands and knees to avoid shock therapy.

It is in reaction to that kind of nonscience that this book is written. There are millions of emotionally sick and mentally twisted people who do need medication and psychiatric care. But there are likewise tens of thousands of physically sick patients who have been told that their illnesses are all in their minds. There are, for instance, thousands of old people suffering only from vitamin deficiency who nonetheless wind up in homes for the senile, where, quite frequently, they are fed atrociously.

In describing those physical disorders which (a) often evade "all the tests" and (b) cause one to be labeled a neurotic, I am *not* writing about exotic and rare conditions, like the tumors of the pancreas that can cause insanity but occur in just a few cases each year. Physicians quickly recognize these conditions. They tend to be less aware of:

*Little Strokes*, which don't paralyze but do cause deterioration of the personality. A tidy person becomes slovenly, a middle-aged man suddenly begins to pursue young girls, a gentle person becomes maniacal, a disciplined mind is no longer able to remember and to concentrate.

*Anxiety, depression, and suicidal tendencies following certain virus infections*, such as influenza, where there is nothing in the life situation or the personality structure to justify the symptoms.

*Allergic reactions*, which don't cause hives, or eczema, or asthma but do change the personality—even to the point of what has been misdiagnosed as "juvenile delinquency" or "adult crime."

*Porphyrinuria*, a physical disease that simulates psychosis or causes the symptoms of neurosis and which is present, undetected, in thousands of patients confined to mental institutions.

*Niacin deficiency*, which in a chronic, mild stage may give rise to symptoms of neurosis or, particularly in older persons, psychosis without causing any of the classic symptoms of vitamin deficiency. (The beginning symptom may be nothing more than gradual loss of a sense of humor!)

*Vitamin B12 deficiency*, which, with no sign of the pernicious anemia it may ultimately cause, may make older people appear senile, with paranoid behavior (delusions of persecution).

*Adrenal gland insufficiency*, which may show itself only as "constitutional inadequacy," or what used to be called "neurasthenia."

*Thyroid gland insufficiency*, which may cause disorientation and confusion, without the weight gain, goiter, or other "classical" symptoms usually characteristic of this condition.

*Multiple sclerosis*, early symptoms of which appear to be purely neurotic, with overtones of hypochondria.

*Malocclusion* (a bad bite), which oddly enough, has been responsible for labeling some people as neurotic.

*Low blood sugar* (functional hypoglycemia), which can masquerade as a hundred physical diseases—from epilepsy to gastric ulcer—and embellish the symptoms with a perfect simulation of neurosis or psychosis.

*Relative dietary deficiency*, in which a person's diet, good enough to meet average needs, falls short of meeting the unusually high requirements with which some people are born, so that a deficiency develops on a "good" diet and creates symptoms indistinguishable from those of emotional or mental disorder.

*Anterior pituitary syndrome*, which is a more exact title for what the medical textbooks mislabel as "constitutional inadequacy," a term that insists that the sufferer is made of stuff too weak to meet the ordinary stresses we all must face and is thereby labeled neurotic, neurasthenic, inadequate, hysterical, ad infinitum, ad nauseam.

*Mercury poisoning*, from the fillings in teeth, which can cause or aggravate symptoms of hypoglycemia, trigger multiple allergies, or cause physical disease.

These disorders share four characteristics:

1. Properly diagnosed, they are usually amenable to treatment.
2. They are often not properly diagnosed.
3. The average "complete physical checkup" misses these disorders.
4. The sufferer is usually and mistakenly given psychotherapy, psychoanalysis, or even shock treatment.

This book has a bias. It leans toward protection of the patient, lost in a medical world he never made.

# 1. For One Person in Every Ten, Sugar Is a Deadly Food, Paving the Way Toward a Hundred Distressing Physical Symptoms, Plus

*All the Tortures of Neurotic and Even Psychotic Behavior. For That Person a Little Sugar Is Akin to a Little Carbolic Acid. If You Are an Average American, You Eat 104 Pounds of Sugar per Year.* \*

Perhaps more than any other disorder, low blood sugar has been responsible for many patients being horizontal on psychiatric couches when they should be vertical at lunch counters.

The medical textbooks call the condition "idiopathic, functional, Seale Harris-type, benign hypoglycemia," which is a physician's way of admitting that the blood sugar is too low to support the nervous system and the brain, and that he doesn't know why. Sometimes, he offers another title for the disorder, one which would seem to be an explanation—"hyperinsulinism." This "explains" the low blood sugar by blaming it on an overactive pancreas. It doesn't tell us, however, why the pancreas is overactive.

Low blood sugar causes an unbelievable array of symptoms. It can make a psychiatric wreck out of a normally well-adjusted individual. It can turn a balanced person into an apprehensive hypochondriac. It creates intolerable anxiety, driving the sufferer to the use of tranquilizers or the ministrations of the psychiatrist. It manufactures unjustified fears, internal feelings of shakiness, and adds intolerable

---

\*Statistics are courtesy of the United States Department of Agriculture. The Carbohydrate Laboratory of the USDA recently tested the tolerance of healthy Americans for the amount of sugar customarily consumed in this country. They found a large percentage of these healthy subjects to react abnormally. The researchers, communicating as concerned private citizens, urged the United States Food and Drug Administration to compel sugar manufacturers to prove that their product is safe.

nightmares to its own kind of insomnia.* The symptoms of low blood sugar not only resemble neurosis or psychosis, they also perfectly imitate or aggravate epilepsy, migraine headache, peptic ulcer, rheumatoid arthritis, juvenile delinquency, insomnia, asthma, and other allergies. Low blood sugar can create some of the "side reactions" blamed on drugs. It can directly cause alcoholism, and could possibly lead to drug addiction.

For all these good reasons, one physician termed low blood sugar what syphilis has been called, "the great imitator," and remarked that any physician who understands this condition, understands all of medicine. He had good reason for the statement, for, himself a victim of hypoglycemia, he had been told erroneously that he could blame his troubles on, variously, brain tumor, diabetes, and neurosis. He was even advised to retire from the practice of medicine, on the grounds that—obviously—he was of stuff too frail to meet the demands made upon a physician.

Like the other disorders dealt with in this book, low blood sugar is too frequently not detected in a "complete medical checkup," and when it is recognized, the treatment prescribed for it (by physicians decades behind the times) is the opposite of what the patient needs; and it makes every symptom worse.

We are all aware that glands may be normal, overactive, or underactive. Most of us know that the underactive thyroid can cause weight gain; the overactive, weight loss and nervousness. Some of us are aware that an overactive pituitary can cause acromegaly. A few may even know that the pancreas is also a gland, and can be underactive, thereby causing diabetes. (*That* is a dangerously oversimplified explanation of what happens.) But few of us have ever given thought to what might happen if the pancreas were *overactive*.

This gland, among other important functions, has the task of producing insulin in amounts geared to the quantity of sugar entering the body. This is the hormone that helps us to burn sugar, and the amount at work in the body is very critical. We realize this as we watch the diabetic giving himself injections of insulin to keep his blood sugar down to normal levels. And we all have heard what happens when a

* In hypoglycemia, the patient does fall asleep, but awakens three or four hours later and can't return to sleep.

diabetic takes a little too much insulin. The effects are dramatic and disquieting—tremor, cold perspiration, dizziness, nervousness, blackout, or even outright unconsciousness. Sometimes, that overdose which lowers the blood sugar too much and too fast is deliberately given, during treatment for mental disease. It is termed "insulin shock treatment."

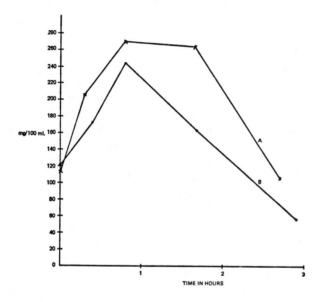

Typical blood sugar curves, showing fasting blood sugar and levels after the administration of sugar as a challenge to the pancreas to determine if it is overresponding and producing excessive amounts of insulin. Note that both tests show that the blood sugar levels, three hours after a dose of sugar, are lower than the original (fasting) level. This is classical low blood sugar.

So, let's speculate now about a condition opposite to diabetes: the pancreas that is overreactive, producing too much insulin. Wouldn't the effect on the sufferer be the same as that of an overdose of insulin on the diabetic? Shock? Dizziness? Nervousness? Cold sweats? Irritability? Shakiness? Anxiety? Even collapse? Of course! And the symptoms would go on and on, for the overdose (overproduction) of insulin would go on and on. A piece of candy or a glass of orange juice (13 percent sugar) will rescue the diabetic from insulin shock. Will it help the person with an overactive pancreas? No—for a very simple reason. The pancreas works because sugar has been eaten. (If it didn't, you'd be diabetic.) If the pancreas is overactive, sugar isn't going to quiet it down; it will stimulate the gland still more. So it is that the person with low blood sugar makes himself worse by eating sugar, and the ironic feature of the disorder is the craving for sweets that accompanies it. Have you ever seen the fat man with the box of candy in his lap, protesting that the more he eats, the more he craves the sweets? He may be telling the truth. He may be a victim of low blood sugar, with obesity as his personal price for it.

The term "hyperinsulinism" really tells much of the story. It defines the pancreas (in low blood sugar) as being overresponsive to sugar. Sweets make it produce more insulin than it should, and it may be so exquisitely reactive to a rise in blood sugar that it may be fooled, literally, into responding—by the sweet taste of saccharin in the mouth, for instance. (Don't be astonished by the hair-trigger mechanism. Did you know that for some people the odor of bacon frying is enough to trigger a gallbladder reaction, and that for others, the *thought* of a favorite food may cause the stomach valve to open?)

All this means that a person with low blood sugar of the type I am describing can be helped only by a diet low in sugar, low in starch (which the body can convert into sugar), and high in the foods that do not "yank" the insulin trigger. These are the fats and the proteins, and such a diet is described in Chapter 9. It isn't only the composition of the diet that matters, but also the timing of the meals. Low blood sugar calls for more frequent refueling than we ordinarily permit ourselves, for our meals are scheduled to conform with the demands of bus and train schedules, rather than physiological requirements.

Now we have a clear view of the hypoglycemic. He tries to function day after day, hour after hour, with some of the symptoms the diabetic briefly endures when he takes an overdose of insulin. He walks around in insulin shock of greater or lesser degree, and this can be, as you will learn, infinitely horrible—all the more so when you don't know what's wrong, can't find out, and wind up diagnosed as a neurotic, hypochondriac, psychotic, eccentric, "nut," or chronic invalid.

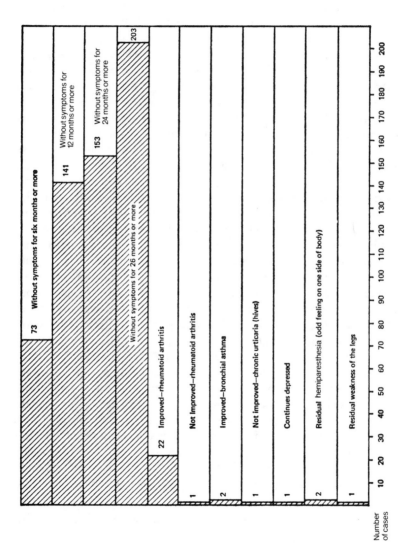

What happened to 600 cases of low blood sugar after treatment.

It must be remembered, too, that man's glands are much like an orchestra. There are rearrangements necessary when one gland suddenly decides to do a solo. Those compensations can be costly. In the case of low blood sugar, the price can include diabetes when the overactive pancreas has exhausted itself.* There are also repercussions from the adreno-sympathetic system; and these can be even more dangerous. They pave the way for what H. Selye called "the stress adaptation syndrome." Of this, more later. You have, at least, been cautioned not to regard hypoglycemia as a minor disruption of the body's economy.

This chapter began by labeling low blood sugar as a disorder of unknown origin. From the preceding discussion of the hair-trigger pancreas and its overproduction of insulin, the cause would seem to be known. Actually, the misbehavior of the gland is a symptom, too, rather than a cause, and we still don't know what makes it go berserk. Good medical textbooks speak of placing the responsibility on an imbalance of the autonomic nervous system—the one that controls those body activities which function without your supervision. That, too, is really not an explanation. We still do not know what causes the imbalance. We *can* try some educated guesses, one of which may startle you, for it places the blame on the genes that came down to us from the Stone Age caveman—a long but logical way to go for an explanation. After all, constitution must play some part in susceptibility to low blood sugar. Otherwise, we'd all suffer from it, since Americans stimulate the pancreas with a teaspoonful of sugar every thirty-five minutes, twenty-four hours a day, for a lifetime. That's perhaps enough sugar to exhaust the pancreas and cause diabetes (which is not proved); it is certainly enough to overstimulate the gland and throw us all into insulin shock. These penalties aren't universal, though we must grant that at least one American man in every four will ultimately reveal signs of a tendency toward diabetes.† But what makes a person susceptible to low blood sugar?

Consider the caveman. Although you are persuaded by television advertising that you will not have enough energy to change channels without a morning cereal that whistles at you from the bowl, the fact is

* "The low blood sugar of today is the diabetes of tomorrow."—Seale Harris, MD.
† E. V. Cowdry, *Problems of Ageing* (Williams and Wilkins, 1943).

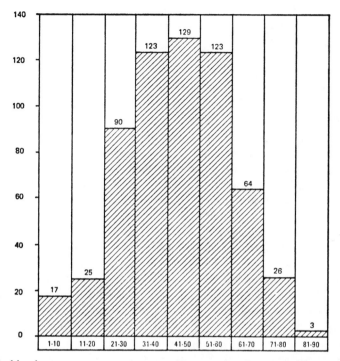

Low blood sugar respects no age group. Here is a distribution of patients by ages (in actual numbers). Note that 21–60 years of age seems to be the chief danger zone.

that the caveman managed to escape the sabertoothed tiger without the benefits of sugar, candy, cold cereal, bread, rice, spaghetti, macaroni, cookies, cakes, barley, corn, and morning porridge. Yet his nervous system and brain required, as ours require, a small, stable supply of sugar for fuel. (That's why low blood sugar has so devastating an impact on personality. The brain reacts promptly and badly to starvation.) Since the caveman lived in an environment that offered practically no concentrated starch or sugar, survival of the fittest created an organism with two characteristics:

1. The body learned to use small amounts of starch and sugar with great efficiency.

2. The body learned to manufacture small (but adequate) amounts of sugar from other types of food—meat, for instance. We still have that ability.

The process of natural selection emphasized a gene that had built-in control of the processes for taking maximum advantage of a very limited supply of sugar. That gene descended through the millennia, and it exists today in some of us, which means that in the twentieth century, the modern caveman, programmed to use only a little starch or sugar with great efficiency, is trying to cope with more than 250 pounds of highly concentrated sugar, flour, and cereals a year. And what are the results? Exhaustion of the pancreas, which tries in vain to produce enough insulin to cope with all that fuel. Overstimulation of the pancreas, driving it into producing more insulin than the body requires. Obesity. It is not by chance that some of these conditions are related. Low blood sugar, increasing the desire for sweets, may of course cause obesity, which in turn is associated with diabetes, which is associated with heart disease and cancer—front-running disorders of our sugar-affluent society. Another pathway to obesity derives from the tendency of hypoglycemics to develop allergies; the allergies in turn can cause fluid retention, making it very difficult to lose weight.

So the survival gene of the caveman, which equipped him to function in an environment with very little concentrated starch and sugar, can have become a lethal gene for modern man, who takes half his calories from carbohydrates—starches and sugars. And one of the consequences could be hypoglycemia.

But there is more than one possible cause. Continued stress can touch off the autonomic nervous system, thereby triggering the pancreas into hyperactivity. The body is not made to withstand "constant stress," a phrase that for the body is a contradiction in terms. Stress is emergency, and emergencies are not constant. The emergency mechanism in the body is built for quick response to temporary crisis. When the crisis becomes permanent, the alarm mechanism breaks down, and degenerative disease results.

Anxiety can touch off low blood sugar, and this is the start of a vicious circle, for low blood sugar causes anxiety. This is part of the mischief that begins when a person with hypoglycemia undergoes psychiatric treatment. Such treatment is in itself a stress and, at least initially, a source of heightened anxiety. Moreover, many times, psychiatric patients, again at least initially, are so emotionally disturbed by the treatment that they either lose interest in food or go to the opposite extreme and nibble constantly. When the overindulgence is in starches and sugars, as it most often is, the hypoglycemic becomes a tragic victim of the "diagnosis by (incomplete) exclusion" that took him to the psychiatric couch.

One variety of low blood sugar arises from and causes monotony, boredom, a sense of aimlessness, and lack of a feeling of achievement. That could describe the situation of many a young executive, lost in the recesses of giant business; and it could be a description, too, of a housewife's reactions to her daily routine.

Stress itself will trigger low blood sugar. It sometimes follows pregnancy and is mistaken then for "childbirth psychosis." It will sometimes be the aftermath of surgery or develop after a long-continued family crisis (the enduring emergency, again). Excessive smoking can start low blood sugar, though in this instance the cure is an immediate halt to smoking. Of all the causes, though, the consumption of more than a hundred pounds of sugar a year looms as the most probable. If you are sure that you don't eat that much, take a look at the chart that follows. Did you know in how many foods sugar is concealed? Did you realize the amounts? For instance, would you eat a portion of apple pie à la mode if you realized that it actually contains 18 teaspoonfuls of sugar? Do not forget that sugar is created by nature, as well as concentrated by man.

APPROXIMATE REFINED CARBOHYDRATE CONTENT OF POPULAR FOODS
EXPRESSED IN AMOUNTS EQUIVALENT TO TEASPOONFULS OF SUGAR
100 grams = 20 teaspoonfuls = 3½ oz. = 400 calories

| FOOD | AMOUNT | SERVING | SUGAR EQUIVALENT |
|---|---|---|---|
| *Candy* | | | |
| Hershey Bar | 60 gm. | 1 bar | 7 tsp. |
| Chocolate cream | 13 gm. | 35 servings to 1 lb. | 2 tsp. |
| Chocolate fudge | 30 gm. | 1½ inches sq. | |
| | | (15 to 1 lb.) | 4 tsp. |
| Chewing gum | | 1 stick | ⅓ tsp. |
| Life saver | | 1 usual size | ⅓ tsp. |

| Food | Amount | Serving | Sugar Equivalent |
|---|---|---|---|
| **Cake** | | | |
| Chocolate cake | 100 gm. | 2-layer, icing (1/12 of cake) | 15 tsp. |
| Angel cake | 45 gm. | 1 pc. (1/12 of large cake) | 6 tsp. |
| Sponge cake | 50 gm. | 1/10 of average cake | 6 tsp. |
| Cream puff (iced) | 80 gm. | 1 average, custard filled | 5 tsp. |
| Doughnut, plain | 40 gm. | 3 inches in diameter | 4 tsp. |
| **Cookies** | | | |
| Macaroons | 25 gm. | 1 large or 2 small | 3 tsp. |
| Gingersnaps | 6 gm. | 1 medium | 1 tsp. |
| Brownies | 20 gm. | 2 × 2 × 3/4 inches | 3 tsp. |
| **Custards** | | | |
| Custard, baked | | 1/2 cup | 4 tsp. |
| Gelatin | | 1/2 cup | 4 tsp. |
| Junket | | 1/8 quart | 3 tsp. |
| **Ice Cream** | | | |
| Ice cream | | 1/8 quart | 5 to 6 tsp. |
| Water ice | | 1/8 quart | 6 to 8 tsp. |
| **Pie** | | | |
| Apple pie | | 1/6 of med. pie | 12 tsp. |
| Cherry pie | | 1/6 of med. pie | 14 tsp. |
| Custard, coconut pie | | 1/6 of med. pie | 10 tsp. |
| Pumpkin pie | | 1/6 of med. pie | 10 tsp. |
| **Sauce** | | | |
| Chocolate, thick | 30 gm. | 1 hp. tsp. | 4½ tsp. |
| Marshmallow | 7.6 gm. | 1 aver. (60 to 1 lb.) | 1½ tsp. |
| **Spreads** | | | |
| Jam | 20 gm. | 1 tbsp. level or 1 hp. tsp. | 3 tsp. |
| Jelly | 20 gm. | 1 tbsp. level or 1 hp. tsp. | 2½ tsp. |
| Marmalade | 20 gm. | 1 tbsp. level or 1 hp. tsp. | 3 tsp. |
| Honey | 20 gm. | 1 tbsp. level or 1 hp. tsp. | 3 tsp. |
| **Milk Drinks** | | | |
| Chocolate (all milk) | | 1 cup, 5 oz. milk | 6 tsp. |
| Cocoa (all milk) | | 1 cup, 5 oz. milk | 4 tsp. |
| Cocomalt (all milk) | | 1 glass, 8 oz. milk | 4 tsp. |
| **Soft Drinks** | | | |
| Coca-Cola | 180 gm. | 1 bottle, 6 oz. | 4⅓ tsp. |
| Ginger ale | 180 gm. | 6 oz. glass | 4⅓ tsp. |

### Cooked Fruits

| | | | |
|---|---|---|---|
| Peaches, canned in syrup | 10 gm. | 2 halves, 1 tbsp. juice | 3½ tsp. |
| Rhubarb, stewed | 100 gm. | ½ cup, sweetened | 8 tsp. |
| Apple sauce (no added sugar) | 100 gm. | ½ cup, scant | 2 tsp. |
| Prunes, stewed, sweetened | 100 gm. | 4 to 5 med., 2 tbsp. juice | 8 tsp. |

### Dried Fruits

| | | | |
|---|---|---|---|
| Apricots, dried | 30 gm. | 4 to 6 halves | 4 tsp. |
| Prunes, dried | 30 gm. | 3 to 4 med. | 4 tsp. |
| Dates, dried | 30 gm. | 3 to 4, stoned | 4½ tsp. |
| Figs, dried | 30 gm. | 1½ to 2 small | 4 tsp. |
| Raisins | 30 gm. | ¼ cup | 4 tsp. |

### Fruits and Fruit Juices

| | | | |
|---|---|---|---|
| Fruit cocktail | 120 gm. | ½ cup, scant | 5 tsp. |
| Orange juice | 100 gm. | ½ cup, scant | 2 tsp. |
| Grapefruit juice, unsweetened | 100 gm. | ½ cup, scant | 2⅓ tsp. |
| Grape juice, commercial | 100 gm. | ½ cup, scant | 3⅓ tsp. |
| Pineapple juice, unsweetened | 100 gm. | ½ cup, scant | 2⅗ tsp. |

Let's return now to the test for low blood sugar. What is it? Why isn't it given as part of the average "complete checkup"? In short, why does low blood sugar evade the physician's probing? When a medical man tests sugar levels in a diabetic's blood, he can use just one drop of blood. Why can't he do that to determine a *deficiency* in blood sugar? Why does low blood sugar evade the examination that is routinely given—in any decent checkup—for diabetes?

From the sugar level in a drop of blood, the medical man can tell whether a person is diabetic. If he is known to be diabetic, the sugar level will tell the physician whether the patient is eating too much sugar and starch and if his insulin dose is high enough. That's all he wants and needs to know. But using such a test for low blood sugar would be completely unsatisfactory. It would be like appraising the efficiency of an automobile motor by checking the fuel in the tank. That would not tell you if the engine runs normally or if it's using fuel excessively. When it is a question of low blood sugar, I am not interested in the amount of blood sugar at a given moment. I want to know what it was before you broke your fast, how much it rose an hour later, and what it was an hour after that. My concern is with the dynamics of your body's handling of sugar, not with the quantity in the blood at a given moment.

So it is that the test for low blood sugar must first be made when the patient has fasted—before breakfast, for instance.* From this first determination of his base level, we can decide if he is producing too much insulin in his sleep. Then he is fed a dose of sugar, and the level in the blood is rechecked at hourly intervals, for as much as six hours.

Normally, after we eat sugar, the blood level rises until insulin is produced; then it levels off and gradually falls until it reaches the fasting level again. In a person with low blood sugar based on an overactive pancreas, any initial rise isn't normal; too much insulin is at work. The rise isn't maintained long enough, again because the insulin response is too great and too prolonged, and, for the same reason, the level drops too rapidly. In fact, in aggravated cases of hypoglycemia, after a dose of sugar the patient may wind up with *less* sugar in his blood than he had when the test started. That's why such patients crave sugar, can't stop nibbling it, and *must* avoid it.

Now that, hopefully, you realize why the conventional test for diabetes will not detect low blood sugar, let's look at two other factors that block its diagnosis. Sometimes, the physician *will* give the long test, with repeated samplings of blood sugar, in a search for early diabetes. Unfortunately, if that test is positive for low blood sugar, and negative, therefore, for diabetes, the delighted physician may completely ignore the positive finding. He is so pleased that his patient doesn't have diabetes that he literally brushes off the significance and importance of the opposite condition—hypoglycemia. After all, it's a malady for which there's a delightful prescription: a candy bar! The second confusing factor can be stated as a truism: one does not find what he is not looking for, and physicians are not low-blood-sugar-minded. This was never more painfully proved than in a report on blood sugars issued by an agency of the United States Public Health Service. The agency was examining patients for diabetes, not for hypoglycemia, by giving the "dual" test: determining the blood sugar level when the patient had fasted, feeding the patient sugar, and then repeating the blood test. In several cases, these tests clearly showed low blood sugar, the second reading being *lower* than the first. The interpretation? In print, the

---

*To ensure an accurate sugar-tolerance test, some physicians precede it with a mandatory three-day high-carbohydrate diet. The author dissents: a carbohydrate load is the mistake in the patient's *accustomed* diet, for which he is paying a price.

researchers said that their technicians must have switched the blood samples, thereby giving the first sugar level as the second, and vice versa! *

This academic tempest in a (sweetened) teapot becomes a very real threat to your well-being, but you are not likely to appreciate that unless you know what low blood sugar can do and what agonies some people have suffered for want of competent diagnosis and treatment. For that reason, out of thousands of patient histories here are three that perfectly illustrate the total impact of hypoglycemia on mind and body. In one case, it made an invalid of a physician. In the second, it forced a wife to work to support her husband for a period of seven years. In the third, it made a secretive alcoholic of a beautiful actress, who then went through four futile years of psychiatric treatment she did not need.

The physician's name—it is given because he himself has printed his own story—was Stephen Gyland. He practiced medicine in Tampa, Florida, until he fell ill. Knowing that a physician is his own worst doctor, he consulted a specialist, hoping for an explanation of his unprovoked anxieties, tremors, weakness, dizziness, faintness, paroxysmal tachycardia (unprovoked rapid beating of the heart), and difficulties with concentration and memory.

The diagnostician told him that he was a neurotic and that these disorders, all in his mind, disqualified him for the practice of medicine. Dr. Gyland refused to accept this verdict and consulted another diagnostician, and then another, until he had visited fourteen specialists and three nationally known diagnostic clinics. He now had an assortment of diagnoses and could take his choice among neurosis, brain tumor, diabetes, and cerebral arteriosclerosis (hardening of the arteries of the brain).

Still sick, still unable to work, still without treatment, Dr. Gyland happened upon the original paper on low blood sugar and its symptoms, published by Seale Harris, MD, in the *Journal of the American Medical Association*, 1924. Here was the diagnosis—here were his symptoms—

* There is a third factor that makes for confusion—*norms* for blood sugar that are *not* normal (see Chapter 7).

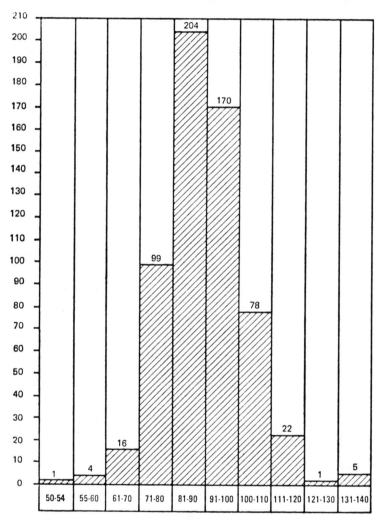

blood sugar level

Variations in fasting blood sugar among 600 patients with low blood sugar. Note that fasting sugar levels *above* what is accepted as the "normal range" are no guarantee that the levels will not drop below normal after the feeding of sugar. Note too that the bulk of these patients fall within the normal range.

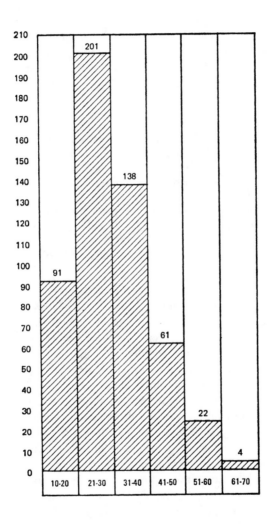

How the six-hour test of tolerance to sugar shows a *drop* below the fasting level after the feeding of sugar to 517 patients. The figures represent the number of patients in each group; the groups are labeled in terms of the amount by which the sugar level in the blood dropped below the fasting level after feeding of sugar.

and here was the treatment (a simple diet). All had been known for some twenty-five years while Gyland wandered from diagnostician to diasnostician, from clinic to clinic! Talk about a cultural lag!

Dr. Gyland took the test for low blood sugar, learned that he had it, went on the appropriate diet, and watched his symptoms fade away. All this makes understandable this portion of a stinging letter he wrote to the *Journal of the American Medical Association* (Vol. 152, July 18, 1953).

> If all physicians would read the work of Dr. Seale Harris . . . thousands of persons would not have to go through what I did. During three years of severe illness, I was examined by fourteen specialists and three nationally known clinics before a diagnosis was made by means of a six-hour glucose (sugar) tolerance test, previous diagnoses having been brain tumor, diabetes, and cerebral arteriosclerosis. . . . Since then I have used this hard-earned knowledge in diagnosis and curing the condition in numerous patients. . . .
>
> (Signed) Stephen Gyland, MD
> Tampa, Florida

Apropos of the physician not finding what he is not looking for, a senior physician at one of the diagnostic clinics made this remark in his newspaper medical column: "I have never seen a case of functional low blood sugar in thirty years of practice." Dr. Gyland, at *that* clinic, was told that he was suffering from a brain tumor!

It is worth noting here that one diagnostician did tell Gyland that he was suffering from low blood sugar, but he prescribed candy bars, which, as you now know, would only worsen his condition.

The blundering of which this physician was the victim is not only still possible—it happens again and again. *You* can be told you're diabetic, as Gyland was, when you're not. *You* can be labeled neurotic when you need diet and vitamins rather than tranquilizers and psychiatrists. *You* can be accused of nonexistent brain tumor or hardening of the arteries of the brain when you should be studying a textbook on nutrition. And if you escape all these errors you may wind up with the correct diagnosis and the wrong treatment, even though Seale Harris, in his pioneering paper in 1924, warned that sugar makes low blood sugar worse.

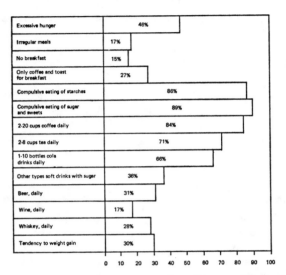

| | |
|---|---|
| Excessive hunger | 46% |
| Irregular meals | 17% |
| No breakfast | 15% |
| Only coffee and toast for breakfast | 27% |
| Compulsive eating of starches | 86% |
| Compulsive eating of sugar and sweets | 89% |
| 2-20 cups coffee daily | 84% |
| 2-8 cups tea daily | 71% |
| 1-10 bottles cola drinks daily | 66% |
| Other types soft drinks with sugar | 36% |
| Beer, daily | 31% |
| Wine, daily | 17% |
| Whiskey, daily | 28% |
| Tendency to weight gain | 30% |

0  10  20  30  40  50  60  70  80  90  100

Percentages of Dr. Gyland's 600 patients with poor eating habits of the type that (a) often reflects low blood sugar, as in the compulsive eating of sweets and starches, and (b) makes low blood sugar worse, as in the drinking of sweetened cola beverages, coffee, tea, and alcohol. These are the worst possible choices for people with hypoglycemia.

Dr. Gyland proved that the alert physician is likely to spot what he suspects, for he went on to treat more than 600 patients for hypoglycemia. Then he wrote a paper about them—the diagnosis, the symptoms, the treatment, and the response. That paper he read before a medical society associated with the American Medical Association, which never printed it in any of their journals. So it was that to study what Dr. Gyland learned from his 600 patients, a Brazilian medical journal had to be consulted and the paper translated from the Portuguese. This may offer a perspective on the blindness of American medicine to hypoglycemia, its prevalence, and what it does to its victims.

It will be revealing to examine the symptoms of which Dr. Gyland's hypoglycemic patients complained and the mistaken diagnoses they had received previously. The following is the list of symptoms; the numbers beside them refer to the percentages of the patients complaining of these particular troubles:

| | |
|---|---|
| Nervousness | 94% |
| Irritability | 89% |
| Exhaustion | 87% |
| Faintness, dizziness, tremor, cold sweats, weak spells | 86% |
| Depression | 77% |
| Vertigo, dizziness | 73% |
| Drowsiness | 72% |
| Headaches | 71% |
| Digestive disturbances | 69% |
| Forgetfulness | 67% |
| Insomnia (awakening and inability to return to sleep) | 62% |
| Constant worrying, unprovoked anxieties | 62% |
| Mental confusion | 57% |
| Internal trembling | 57% |
| Palpitation of heart, rapid pulse | 54% |
| Muscle pains | 53% |
| Numbness | 51% |
| Indecisiveness | 50% |
| Unsocial, asocial, antisocial behavior | 47% |
| Crying spells | 46% |
| Lack of sex drive (females) | 44% |
| Allergies | 43% |
| Incoordination | 43% |
| Leg cramps | 43% |
| Lack of concentration | 42% |
| Blurred vision | 40% |
| Twitching and jerking of muscles | 40% |
| Itching and crawling sensations on skin | 39% |
| Gasping for breath | 37% |
| Smothering spells | 34% |
| Staggering | 34% |
| Sighing and yawning | 30% |
| Impotence (males) | 29% |

| | |
|---|---|
| Unconsciousness | 27% |
| Night terrors, nightmares | 27% |
| Rheumatoid arthritis | 24% |
| Phobias, fears | 23% |
| Neurodermatitis | 21% |
| Suicidal intent | 20% |
| Nervous breakdown | 17% |
| Convulsions | 2% |

The patients also commented on changes in personality in the form of unaccustomed lapses in moral conduct, carelessness in dress, and tendencies to drug and alcohol addiction.

Look back over that list of symptoms. How could these patients have convinced any physician that they weren't neurotics?

A large percentage of them *had* been told that their symptoms were expressions of neurotic conflicts. Here are some of the mistaken diagnoses they received before Dr. Gyland subjected them to the simple but time-consuming sugar-tolerance test:

Mental retardation
Neurosis
"Slightly nervous"
Chronic urticaria (hives)
Neurodermatitis (itching, rash, from "nervous" causes)
Meniere's syndrome (loss of hearing, dizziness associated with it, and noises in the ears)
Cerebral arteriosclerosis
Cephalagia, hemicrania (pain in the head or in half the head)
Psychoneuroticism
Chronic bronchial asthma
Rheumatoid arthritis
Parkinson's syndrome (senile palsy)
Paroxysmal tachycardia (rapid beating of the heart)
"Imaginary sickness"
Menopause
Alcoholism
Diabetes

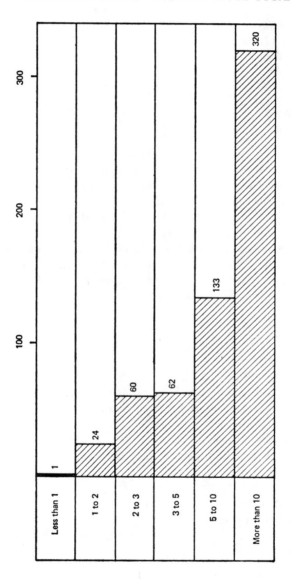

The number of years Gyland's patients suffered before their low blood sugar was recognized and properly treated.

Hyperinsulinism (the correct diagnosis—but treated with candy bars!)

The second history is brief, but no less poignant a record of medical blindness to hypoglycemia. The patient was a stationary engineer, who was forced, as a semi-invalid, to retire from his profession. He had had a series of blackouts, interspersed with episodes of "gray-outs," during which he was not unconscious but could not control his movements and was not able to make himself understood. Because his work involved moving machinery, he was a hazard to himself and to his employer, and on the advice of his doctor, who labeled him an odd type of epileptic, since the brain waves did *not* spell out epilepsy, he remained at home for seven years, afraid even to venture into the streets for fear that he might hurt himself with a sudden fall.

During those years, his wife went to work and supported the household. No attempt was made to check the diagnosis until, by pure chance, the patient tuned in a network broadcast in which I was interviewing Dr. Herman Goodman, of New York City, who originated a short test for hypoglycemia that much reduces the expense (and the time) needed to establish the diagnosis. The patient called this physician, underwent the test, and was found to have blood sugar levels so low that it was amazing that he managed ever to remain on his feet. He is now well—as long as he avoids the concentrated starches and sugar—and back at work.

The third history concerns a show girl, nearly six feet tall, who, years before, had been one of Billy Rose's "long-stemmed roses." Though a happy wife and mother, she found herself so weak and apathetic, particularly in the morning hours, that shortly after pregnancy (the trigger, again!) she began secretive drinking, which progressed into outright alcoholism. This she somehow concealed from her husband, but she did go to her physician, who counseled her, and, after a "complete physical checkup," prescribed a stimulant and, on the familiar basis of diagnosis by exclusion, sent her to a psychiatrist. Four years of psychiatric treatment made the doctor more affluent, but the patient remained an alcoholic. Then came the morning that, as she described it, she was too weak to turn off the radio when her little boy switched it on and, as a captive audience, she found herself listening to the author,

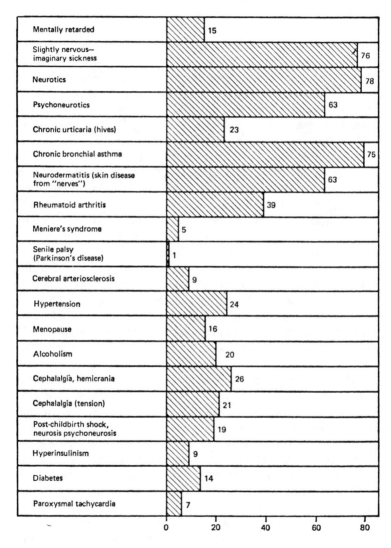

| | |
|---|---|
| Mentally retarded | 15 |
| Slightly nervous— imaginary sickness | 76 |
| Neurotics | 78 |
| Psychoneurotics | 63 |
| Chronic urticaria (hives) | 23 |
| Chronic bronchial asthma | 75 |
| Neurodermatitis (skin disease from "nerves") | 63 |
| Rheumatoid arthritis | 39 |
| Meniere's syndrome | 5 |
| Senile palsy (Parkinson's disease) | 1 |
| Cerebral arteriosclerosis | 9 |
| Hypertension | 24 |
| Menopause | 16 |
| Alcoholism | 20 |
| Cephalalgia, hemicrania | 26 |
| Cephalalgia (tension) | 21 |
| Post-childbirth shock, neurosis psychoneurosis | 19 |
| Hyperinsulinism | 9 |
| Diabetes | 14 |
| Paroxysmal tachycardia | 7 |

Breakdown of previous diagnoses (except for nine cases correctly diagnosed as hypoglycemia but treated with sugar!).

deep in a discussion of low blood sugar as a pathway to alcoholism. She wrote for literature, consulted her physician and demanded—which she had to—a glucose-tolerance test. This confirmed her hypoglycemia. To her delight, after six or seven weeks of the proper diet, she found her desire for alcohol diminishing. Eventually, she stopped drinking entirely, her energy reserves rebuilt, and she was able to terminate the psychiatric treatment.

You have now read a very few of the stories of 603 people, including Gyland's patients, who know what idiopathic, functional hypoglycemia can do to body and mind and who are painfully aware that many American medical men are painfully unaware that this is a common disorder that masquerades as half a hundred other diseases. They know, those who have walked this painful path, that sugar may be described as an "energy food" for millions of people, but for them it is the way to dysfunction of the body, dislocation of the mind, and disturbances of the relationship between the two.

## 2. Low Blood Sugar Causes "Neurosis"; Neurosis Causes Low Blood Sugar

A high index of suspicion has its corollary, of course, which is the possibility of obsession. It is not uncommon among medical men. One practitioner has in print declared his conviction that daily high colonics are a sovereign remedy for most of the ills to which the flesh falls prey. The results he reports do not include the paralysis of the rectal muscles that developed in some patients, for which they had to be treated before normal, unassisted elimination could be restored. Another physician believes that enlarged prostates are responsible for virtually all the complaints of older men, so that in his office no geriatric male patient escapes digital prostate massage.

What is the possibility that Dr. Gyland, under the impact of his own troubles with hypoglycemia, went beyond a high index of suspicion and managed to find hypoglycemia where it didn't exist or blamed it for symptoms it didn't cause? That question occurred to a psychiatrist who was willing to accept low blood sugar as a simulator of neurosis or even psychosis, but found it difficult to understand why Gyland's low blood sugar should have been confused with brain tumor, diabetes, and cerebral arteriosclerosis.

He is Dr. Harry Salzer, psychiatrist, who not only came to appreciate the many faces of hypoglycemia—particularly in his own field—but the ease with which it may be confused with other disease entities. He was greatly impressed by what he learned from experience with his own psychiatric patients when he searched for low blood sugar and, finding it, treated it dietetically; so much so that he later became medical director of a foundation dedicated to research in hypoglycemia.

Dr. Salzer, after reading the medical literature on hypoglycemia of the functional type—including at least one paper that insists that the condition is so rare as to be virtually nonexistent—began his own research by watching during the course of his practice for symptoms of possible low blood sugar. The title of the report he ultimately published is in itself an affirmation of what Gyland said about nervous disorders caused by hypoglycemia: "Functional Hyperinsulinism as a Cause of Neuro-Psychiatric Illness."

In this paper, Dr. Salzer remarks that in 1953 he began to search for symptoms of hypoglycemia in his patients and turned up one verified case. In 1954, he identified eight cases; in 1955, eleven. Finally, it became apparent to him that "this condition was present and unrecognized in hundreds of patients." In 1956, he justified that statement by demonstrating the presence of low blood sugar in 87 of the 216 patients he examined and treated in his private practice, and this impelled him to go back to patients he had previously examined and treated in the years before his index of suspicion for low blood sugar had risen; and he candidly admits that well over a hundred cases of hypoglycemia had evaded his prior examinations in that group.

His patients profited from his change in perspective. He tells the story, for instance, of a young man who was hospitalized because he was depressed, suicidal, and dangerously hostile: he had, in fact, tried to choke his own mother. With five electric shock treatments* he im-

---

* It is my opinion that electric and insulin shock therapies are atavisms, returns to the snakepits into which our superstitious forefathers dropped their insane in the hope that the horror would drive the "devils" out of the psychotic skull. Speculate on what might happen if insulin shock treatment is applied to a patient already suffering from the effects of overproduction of the hormone. One expert who was asked this question said flatly that death could result. One case is known that at least in part indicates the impact of such a gratuitously added insult as insulin dosage piled upon hyperinsulinism. The patient was an elderly woman who, when first treated with insulin shock went into convulsions so violent that a spinal injury resulted, a mishap that forced her to wear a back brace for the rest of her days. She was later subjected to new administerings of the treatment when she, at certain intervals, again lapsed into incoherency and disorientation. While in the hospital in what proved to be the last of her relapses and awaiting the start of the shock treatments, she happened upon one of my broadcasts on functional hypoglycemia and was startled to realize that she had all the symptoms of low blood sugar—from the craving for sweets to the anxiety and the wide-eyed wakefulness after a half-night's sleep. Her physician was outraged by her self-diagnosis on the basis of what he termed "radio quackery" and refused to administer the glucose-tolerance test she was doggedly demanding. She persisted until she got it, although she was forced to change doctors in the process. Hypoglycemia was clearly indicated, and, with adherence to the right diet, she was able to spend her remaining years as a normal, balanced, mentally alert person.

proved slightly, but a month later, it became necessary to give him five more. This series brought improvement that lasted for about nine months, after which the patient, observing his symptoms returning, became convinced himself that he was again becoming psychotic. This time his condition was diagnosed as "schizo-affective psychosis"—a dreadful label, signifying a mental disorder for which there is really no known cause and little satisfactory treatment, and which has been responsible for the institutionalization of tens upon tens of thousands of patients.

But Dr. Salzer, his clinical eye now directed toward hypoglycemia, insisted on obtaining an accurate record of this patient's dietary habits, from which emerged a history of an endless intake of sweets, potatoes, bread, pie, cake and the inevitable coffee and cola drinks. A six-hour glucose-tolerance test was performed, which, consistent with such a dietary record, showed clear evidence of low blood sugar. The condition was promptly treated with the conventional hypoglycemia diet. The patient's subsequent comment is revealing and succinct: "I am better," he marveled, "than I have been in years." The reader here may speculate on the difficulty of persuading such a patient or his family or, possibly, his family doctor that a mere diet could bring such dramatic change in personality, mental function, and approach to interpersonal relationships!

The young man was, of course, spared further shock treatments, and a follow-up check, some two and a half years later, found the patient completely well.

It is disconcerting to speculate on such a patient's fate if he had— like so many mentally diseased persons—been confined in an institution. We are all familiar with the diets supplied in many mental hospitals, where food budgets dictate that cheap starches and sugars be the mainstay of the diet; where, even if the food were essentially good and the menus properly balanced, the exigencies of mass food preparation and the shortages of skilled kitchen help would combine to make the meals unpalatable; and where similar shortages of professional personnel make it impossible routinely to screen patients for such disorders as hypoglycemia (if, indeed, the psychiatric staff could be wooed away from chemotherapy long enough to focus their attention on such time-consuming considerations as six-hour glucose-tolerance tests, high pro-

tein meals, and proper between-meal feedings). Add to this
lem that institutional life must depress sugar curves, as Dr. Sydney A.
Portis' work, quoted later, implies, and you can see how unpromising
the future is for a hypoglycemic mistakenly confined in an institution.
And the visiting relatives, bearing the usual candy and cookies, would
offer nothing but aggravation of such a patient's condition!

Another of the Salzer patient histories tells the story of a forty-nine-
year-old woman who had been subjected to two unnecessary operations
for persistent headaches over the right eye and pain in the eye itself,
both, it later appeared, caused by hypoglycemia.* The pain, of course,
survived the surgery and persisted until she was tested and treated for
hypoglycemia, when all symptoms disappeared. The overlooked clues
to low blood sugar included episodes of unprovoked sweating, insomnia, cold hands and feet, spontaneous tachycardia, and heart palpitation, all complicated by the malaise so characteristic of hypoglycemia.
Her dietary history, though suggestive, was neglected, too: a breakfast
of coffee, cola drinks for lunch, and, for TV snacks, peanut brittle and
as much as a pint of ice cream. Ice cream is 16 percent sugar, but for
some hypoglycemics, the large amount of fat in this favorite American
dish slows the absorption of sugar so much that they are able to tolerate
it. See page 171 for a discussion of a similar effect of fiber, such as bran.

In the fourth hour of the glucose-tolerance test, her blood sugar
dropped to 25, a level lower than any the physician had previously
encountered. Interestingly, the blood sugar level at the end of the third
hour was so high that diabetes could have been diagnosed, and had the
test been terminated then—as thousands of such tests are—that would
have been the justified conclusion. The later appearance of low blood
sugar, of course, makes this the classic example of dysinsulinism, the
paradox that allows a person to be both diabetic and hypoglycemic and
in which a dose of sugar initially elicits a sluggish, diabetic-type of
insulin production by the pancreas, but in the later hours, makes the
insulin level rise sharply, causing low blood sugar. This has been found

---

* Medically trained readers should know that she had been diagnosed as suffering from temporal arteritis and cervical arthritis, for which she underwent
sectioning of the right temporal artery and a cervical hemilaminectomy for
removal of bone spurs thought to cause the pain by impinging on nerve root
foramina!

to be the explanation when diabetics develop another disease, such as asthma, against which high blood sugar is ordinarily a protection. It also explains the occasional instances of severe shock when a diabetic takes his accustomed dose of insulin and reacts excessively, the dose undoubtedly having coincided with one of his periods of hypoglycemia. All this emphasizes the importance of the full six-hour glucose-tolerance test and the possible inadequacies of the short method described in Chapter 7. If, for instance, any short test should argue for normal blood sugar or for diabetes, and yet the symptoms point clearly toward hypoglycemia, the competent physician will extend the test, remembering that it is used only to *confirm* the diagnosis, which he himself must *make.*

Dr. Salzer, then, found himself in complete agreement with the medical men whose research in hypoglycemia preceded his, particularly, in his own field of psychiatry. Gyland had remarked: "Harris verified that [in hypoglycemia] the neurological symptoms are common: [E. M.] Abrahamson found a great number of cases of functional hyperinsulinism in hospitals for psychiatry. Of our cases, 236 had been classified before as 'slightly nervous,' 'imaginarily sick,' 'neurotic,' or 'psychoneurotic'; in 19, the troubles had appeared after childbirth, some, six months before, others, twelve years before. In 78 cases, psychotherapy was applied, and in 32, convulsotherapy with electric shocks, without results. In three patients, it was necessary for a complete recovery to apply psychotherapy after the cure of hyperinsulinism." Then, significantly, Gyland added: "After seeing all those nervous ruins regain health, I do not think it is necessary for anybody to learn to live with his nerves."

Salzer's conclusions are fit and logical: "A six-hour glucose-tolerance test and careful dietary history, particularly about the ingestion of starches, sweets, and intake of caffeine, are considered indispensable for any patient presenting himself for neuro-psychiatric examination. By making the diagnosis of functional hyperinsulinism and teaching patients what they should eat, many will be spared years of suffering, unnecessary operations, electro-shock therapy, and the hazards inherent in taking sedatives, stimulants, and tranquilizers." Who could disagree?

How a hypoglycemic finds himself labeled as neurotic or psychotic is well illustrated in the histories Salzer gives of 200 of his patients with low blood sugar. His table of the previous (and erroneous) diagnoses somewhat resembles Gyland's, with differences attributable to Salzer's field, psychiatry, which would lead one to expect that the large majority of his patients were sent to him because of what appeared to be purely emotional or mental disorders. And so it was: thirty-eight of them had been diagnosed as suffering from "psychoneurotic depression." Thirty-three were said to be suffering from depressive reaction." Six had been accused of paranoid schizophrenia, a dreadful diagnosis if one remembers that Freud considered all paranoids to be latent homosexuals, and that schizophrenia with orthodox treatment has a gloomy prognosis. Four more had been told they had undifferentiated schizophrenia, and two were tagged with "schizo-affective psychosis," the diagnosis of the young man whose story was told in detail earlier in this chapter. Manic-depressive psychosis had been the decision in four cases, and postpartum (after childbirth) depression was supposed to be the illness of two women. A grab-bag title of "psychopathic personality" had been used to describe the symptoms of three cases. Marriage also came in for its share of the purported blame: three were allegedly victims of "marital maladjustment," which brings to mind the marriage counselor who insists that battling spouses both undergo glucose-tolerance tests. * Finally, in the category of psychiatric diagnosis, there were nine cases of chronic alcoholism.

Physical diagnoses, involving the nervous system, were made of 38 patients. Thirteen were previously told they had convulsive disorders of several types. Six were assured that they suffered from headaches of "unknown origin," something the patients themselves could have discerned without medical aid. Five were assured that their pains came from a physical entity—cervical root syndrome, and five more were horrified by diagnoses of multiple sclerosis. Migraine, narcolepsy, posttraumatic encephalopathy (brain pathology due to injury), probable Huntington's chorea (a hereditary predisposition toward a variety of St. Vitus), and torticollis (wryneck) covered the remaining nine diagnoses

---

* The tensions of a marriage need not be caused by hypoglycemia, but they can cause it and be worsened by it. The wife who rushes to get her husband his breakfast because "before it he's impossible" may be more perceptively diagnostic than she knows.

in this group. All the other patients—fifteen—were assigned such disorders as menopause, hypertensive cardiovascular disease (heart and blood vessel disorders associated with high blood pressure), neurodermatitis (skin disorders with a neurological basis), and hypothyroidism.

It must be made plain, in summarizing this tragedy of medical misjudgment, that some of these diagnoses may have been correct. An underactive thyroid, for instance, could have been present and responsible for some of the symptoms of the patients labeled hypothyroid; but it wasn't the dominant cause of their troubles. How far afield these diagnoses went may be judged by Salzer's own tabulation of results achieved by treating these people with the diet for hypoglycemia: of 200 patients, 80 recovered completely, and 75 were greatly improved. Of this total of 155 patients, all who stayed with the diet have remained well. Before treatment with the hypoglycemic diet, 36 patients in this group of 200 had received electric shock treatment. That 18 percent dropped to 9.5 percent who needed such treatment after following the hypoglycemia diet. In addition to this almost 50 percent drop in the number considered to need this drastic treatment, there was also a reduction in frequency. A patient who had required fifteen shock treatments to recover from a previous depressive episode, now needed only three, and the same degree of benefit was constant for others suffering from depression.

These patients, contrary to what one might expect, did not all show signs of severe hypoglycemia. About 8 percent of them, in the six-hour test, showed a drop of only 10 to 20 milligrams (mgs.) percent below the original fasting blood sugar levels, thereby fitting into the type described by Gyland as "pre-hypoglycemic." Despite the mildness of their hypoglycemia, this group responded to the diet by a complete recovery or at least a great improvement in their conditions.

It is important to remember Dr. Salzer's conclusions, so that you may resort to them when you meet, as you will, psychologists and psychiatrists as well as general practitioners who tend to forget that *psychosomatic* is a word that has its reverse: *somatopsychic*. "Unquestionably," said Dr. Salzer, "functional hyperinsulinism is an important cause of neuro-psychiatric illness." Anticipating the demand for a quantitative evaluation of "important cause," Dr. Salzer added, "A figure near 40 percent will represent the approximate frequency with which functional hyperinsulinism should be found in neuro-psychiatric practice."

Forty percent! Four patients in ten, who face deep, probing psychoanalysis, deep or superficial psychotherapy, conditioned reflex therapy, nondirective therapy, chemotherapy, tranquilizers, psychoenergizers, sedatives, shock therapy, or even institutionalization, when what they need is a proper diet!

This is why I have said that there are patients horizontal on psychiatric couches who should be vertical at lunch counters. And it does seem a gratuitous insult that among the effects of psychological treatment there is often (in the early stages, at least) a muddying of the mental and the emotional waters, concomitant with a loss of interest in food, a nervous nibbling of carbohydrates, or bizarre distortions of the daily menu—attacks on the nutritional well-being of the patient that must inevitably worsen hypoglycemia. It must also be remembered that this condition is not merely a shifting in the dynamics of the body's management of sugar, but must also involve changes in liver function. The liver is slow to express insult, but it is an organ that is even slower to respond to a more favorable treatment.

These data have been drawn from Dr. Salzer's paper, read before the Section of Nervous and Mental Diseases at the meeting of the American Medical Association, June 1957. We know about his later experience with hypoglycemia, for the psychiatrist delivered another report before the National Medical Association, in August 1965, by which time he had treated more than 300 hypoglycemic patients. In the later paper, we are given a list of psychiatric and neurologic symptoms that overlap those of Gyland's patients and add a few new ones. They are listed below, along with the percentages of patients complaining of them:

| | |
|---|---|
| Depression | 60% |
| Insomnia | 50% |
| Anxiety | 50% |
| Irritability | 45% |
| Crying spells | 32% |
| Phobias | 31% |
| Difficulty in concentration | 30% |

| | |
|---|---|
| Confusion | 26% |
| Unsocial or antisocial behavior | 22% |
| Restlessness | 20% |
| Suicidal tendencies | 10% |

Before I proceed to Salzer's list of his patients' neurological symptoms, it might be instructive to remove one or two of these symptoms from this cold and dispassionate listing and demonstrate to you what they did to just one person. The subject was a clerical worker in a large city, employed in a responsible position by a major radio station. She found herself depressed and, on several occasions, suicidal, symptoms that no one knew about except herself and her general practitioner. She had an obvious excuse for the depression and the drive toward self-destruction in that she had, on a number of occasions and without apparent provocation, burst into tears, which she could not hide, as she had hidden her depression, from her fellow workers. She was filled with fears, among them a claustrophobia that made it almost impossible for her to ride the subway to work or to take the elevator to her floor. Her greatest fear was a rational one, the fear that the company would fire her before she was eligible for her pension. She was "medicated" for her complaints, but her symptoms grew steadily worse, until she was tested and treated for hypoglycemia. She has been symptom-free for more than ten years, occasional deviations from the diet in the early days of therapy having taught her that for her a little sugar is indeed like a little carbolic acid.

The neurological symptoms of Salzer's patients included:

| | |
|---|---|
| Headache | 45% |
| Vertigo | 42% |
| Tremor | 38% |
| Muscle pains and backache | 33% |
| Numbness | 29% |
| Blurred vision | 24% |
| Muscular twitching or cramps | 23% |
| Staggering | 18% |
| Fainting or blackouts | 14% |
| Convulsions | 14% |

Physical complaints included:

| | |
|---|---|
| Exhaustion | 67% |
| Sweating | 41% |
| Tachycardia (unprovoked rapid beating of the heart) | 37% |
| Anorexia (significant loss of appetite) | 32% |
| Chronic indigestion | 29% |
| Cold hands or feet | 26% |
| Joint pain | 23% |
| Obesity | 19% |
| Abdominal spasms | 16% |

At this point, the reader should refer to the title of the paper in which these statistics were presented—"Functional Hyperinsulinism as a Cause of Neuro-Psychiatric Illness"—to be reminded that these symptoms were attributed to purely psychic, purely emotional causes. It is necessary to reemphasize that every patient who is suspected of neurosis or psychosis must be given the benefit of the doubt, must receive a sugar-tolerance test—the six-hour method, preferably. If the short method is used, it must be followed by the longer test if there is any doubt. Four in every ten—if Salzer's estimate is accurate, and there is no reason, with the size of the group on which he bases it, why it should not be—will be found to have hypoglycemia, a finding that for these victims opens the door to great relief or total cure. And if it should be necessary to continue the diet for a lifetime, as may be the case, is this a bad exchange for shock therapy, psychotherapy, psychoanalysis, hypnosis, and a prolonged dependence on the tranquilizer, psychoenergizer, and sleeping pill? You must remember that side reactions to a number of tranquilizers are so devastating that clinics have actually been organized for the sole purpose of attempting to treat these adverse reactions. Is not the time, effort, and money wasted on six negative tests in every ten justified by the escape of four in every ten from the twilight zone of existing rather than living?

A psychologist has said that the preceding brings up two provocative questions. First, how do you distinguish a "genuine" neurotic from a hypoglycemic without a sugar-tolerance test? (He could have had a bias; the psychologist is not a medical man, can not, himself, legally perform or order such a test.) His second question dealt with high blood sugar: does it, he wondered, protect against symptoms of neurosis? The first query is based on an assumption that is fallacious: not only are hypoglycemic symptoms of neurosis identical with and indistinguishable from those caused by purely emotional stress, but many "genuine" neurotics have low blood sugar as a complication of their emotional disorder. His second question invites a close look at diabetics to determine if they show any particular immunity to symptoms of neurosis.

There are some specialists in psychosomatic medicine who believe that most diabetics have disturbed personalities, but diabetic specialists almost universally complain that the sangfroid of their patients is a distinct problem, for it is most difficult to persuade such phlegmatic people that their health and their lives depend on their faithfulness to the instructions they are given, which they and they alone can carry out.

So it is that anyone who pursues the assumption that high blood sugar protects against neurotic behavior will find himself both supported and opposed. After all, there is little awareness of the opposite thesis, to which I have devoted so much research, that low blood sugar can perfectly masquerade as neurosis. This, despite the fact that hyperinsulinism was recognized in 1924—more than sixty years ago! This, despite the warnings given even by conservative authorities in medicine, such as encyclopedias like *Oxford Looseleaf Medicine*, which remarks: "Hypoglycemia as a disease entity should be kept in mind by all physicians. . . . The attacks may suggest epilepsy, acute alcoholism, or some functional disorder, such as hysteria. It is for these reasons that patients with hypoglycemia are frequently referred to neurological or psychiatric clinics." The admonition was lost on a medical profession dominated by the philosophy that Walter Alvarez, of the Mayo Clinic, expressed when he said that in some thirty years of practice he had never seen a case of functional hyperinsulinism. He *had*, of course, seen the organic type, caused by a growth in the pancreas. So it was that surgeons enthusiastically operated upon patients with hyperinsulinism, and when they failed to find the expected tumor of the pancreas, they did not permit this absence to destroy the theory that low blood sugar is always of organic origin. They simply concluded that the tumor was there, but too small to be seen! We might at this point remember that among the patients with unrecognized functional hypoglycemia who visited the Mayo Clinic was Dr. Gyland himself.

Aware of this philosophy, two physicians—R. H. Hoffman and E. M. Abrahamson—decided on an experiment that might shake up entrenched indifference to the role of functional hypoglycemia as a simulator of neurosis. Their idea had an appealing simplicity: they proposed to give a six-hour glucose-tolerance test to 220 patients who had been diagnosed as neurotic, and were genuinely so, but who also had certain physical symptoms that suggested the possibility of low blood sugar. And so it proved; many of them did in fact have hypoglycemia, and when this was brought under control, three dividends accrued. The physical symptoms faded; the "genuinely" neurotic symptoms also lessened; and the patients, feeling better on both counts, became more amenable to psychiatric treatment.

Having demonstrated that hypoglycemia may be a complication of genuine neurosis in patients who show physical symptoms of low blood sugar, Hoffman and Abrahamson now extended their investigation to neurotics with no physical complaints suggesting hypoglycemia. These patients, unlike the first group, had no craving for sweets, no omnipresent fatigue, no blackouts, but of course had the full panoply of neurotic complaints—depressions, fears, compulsions. The six-hour glucose-tolerance test in this group revealed an astonishing incidence of mild hypoglycemia, and—unexpectedly—the diet helped these people with their purely emotional symptoms quite as much as it had aided those in the first group.

The first group—patients who were neurotic but who had physical signs of low blood sugar—numbered 220, of whom 205 were found to be suffering from hypoglycemia; and all improved with the dietary treatment. The second experiment, involving neurotic patients with no physical signs of hypoglycemia, ultimately encompassed nearly 700, more than 600 of whom proved to have low blood sugar and similarly responded to dietary therapy. What is astonishing is not the percentage of neurotics—with or without physical symptoms of hypoglycemia—who proved to have low blood sugar, nor the percentage whose physical and emotional symptoms improved as they changed their diets. What is astonishing is that this information is astonishing today, when Harris in

*1936*, writing in the *Annals of Internal Medicine*, made this remark: "nervous syndromes [groups of symptoms] such as psychasthenia, neurasthenia, muscular asthenia, migraine, petit mal, narcolepsy, epilepsy, and psychosis" are among the "varied and fantastic" ways in which hypoglycemia can distort human function. He referred to neurasthenia, which is a discarded term whose definition may prove interesting in the light of what the reader has just encountered. A medical dictionary of that day defined it as causing "lack of energy, abnormal fatigue, reluctance to participate in activity, pain in the back, insomnia, a sense of fullness after eating, digestive complaints, and palpitation of the heart." Surely, some of the people with these symptoms were actually suffering from hypoglycemia, and it is interesting, now that we have some understanding of the condition, to look back across the decades and survey the treatment for "neurasthenia." It consisted of having the patient bedded, usually in a sanitarium, in an atmosphere of peace— with drawn shades, tiptoeing attendants, soothing baths, bed rest, and absolute quiet. To this shielding from the noise, confusion, and stress of everyday living, much of his recovery was attributed, but in those days of blissful ignorance of vitamin deficiencies or hypoglycemia, one aspect of the therapy was never given credit: the patient was fed nourishing, frequent, and regular meals. If his condition was the result in whole or in part of imbalanced meals, the treatment was certainly bound to help him!

Up to now we have discussed hypoglycemia caused by a pancreas made overactive by tension, by improper diet, and, rarely, by a pancreatic tumor. We have learned that there is little point in discussing the *severity* of low blood sugar, because big troubles can result from little deficits in it.* There remain some other causes of hypoglycemia with which the reader should be acquainted. Drug-induced low blood sugar is possible. Vitamin deficiency—especially in B Complex vitamins— can disturb carbohydrate metabolism, particularly via changes in liver function, and contribute to hypoglycemia. That is why the excessive

---

* There are people with mild hypoglycemia who have severe symptoms, and some with severe hypoglycemia whose symptoms are comparatively mild. There are patients with hypoglycemia who have no symptoms at all. Others have clear-cut symptoms of low blood sugar, with "normal" blood sugar levels. Some of these contradictions are discussed in Chapter 7, "Abnormal Norms."

intake of sweets characteristic of hypoglycemics invites the use of supplements of Vitamin B Complex, to make sure that liver function is not disturbed. Because these supplements are aimed at helping liver function, they should not be chosen at random. It is necessary to find a Vitamin B Complex concentrate that supplies a significant amount of choline and inositol. A satisfactory supplementary supply of these two factors, which often are not present in concentrates in adequate amounts, would be 1000 mgs. of choline and 500 of inositol in the recommended daily dose. If you cannot locate a Vitamin B Complex preparation complying with this stipulation, it is possible to buy choline and inositol, separately tableted or combined in one tablet. In some formulae, methionine is also added. This is desirable, since methionine also helps liver function. This type of Vitamin B Complex is as important to hypoglycemics as is the consistent use of the chromium glucose-tolerance factor. The type I prefer is concentrated from yeast, for metallic chromium may not be efficiently utilized; indeed, failure to manufacture this factor from chromium in the body can be part of the problem in both hypoglycemia and diabetes. The chromium glucose-tolerance factor usually is supplied in 100 mcgs. concentration, and I employ from one to two tablets daily. You should also remember that low blood sugar can be a result of faulty absorption of sugar, a condition helped by the same type of dietary treatment and vitamin supplementation used for hyperinsulinism.

There is, though, a type of low blood sugar that differs from the others. Its root cause is an emotional disturbance, and its characteristic is a "flat glucose-tolerance curve." The term "flat" seems paradoxical when used to modify "curve," but it will prove apt when it is examined. This is the disturbance in sugar metabolism that comes about when a person is, for instance, forced into an occupation in which he finds neither zest nor challenge. The tension is low-grade; so is the upset in the dynamics of the management of blood sugar. Here we are dealing with a low-key hypoglycemia of a special type, different from that we have been discussing and unrelated to the very mild type of low blood sugar which Gyland characterized as "pre-hypoglycemic."

These sufferers are described as showing a "flat sugar-tolerance curve," but the medical term is dry and undramatic, giving no indication of the impact of chronic low-grade cerebral starvation, which is what the term actually implies. The deficit in fuel for the brain and nervous system is not great enough to yield the dramatic symptoms of hypoglycemia. Their chief complaint, as Portis aptly quotes it, is "pernicious inertia." This is the common denominator in patients with a flat curve: their lives are equally flat, uninteresting, without challenge, without zest. Their occupations are distasteful to them, forced upon them by circumstances beyond their control, and they react, to quote Portis, with "apathy, loss of zest, a general letdown feeling of aimlessness, a revulsion against the routine of everyday life, be it occupational activity or household duties."

Portis makes it clear that he considers this condition to be an apt example of the influence of mind on body. One of his papers on it, for that reason, was delivered before the American Psychosomatic Society. In his eight years of study of this type of disturbance of the blood sugar, he became convinced that the flat curve results when a person finds no challenge and no sense of achievement in pursuing his (inescapable) duties; and the body responds to the deficit in mental and emotional challenge by *not* attuning itself to the demands made upon it, with the result that there is an imbalance created between the function of the adrenal glands, which elevate blood sugar, and the pancreas, which lowers it. This results in a chronic half-starvation of the brain. The sugar levels in the blood do not dip low enough to cause blackout, nor rise high enough to permit efficient function, and the person is only half-alive, existing in a twilight zone where constant fatigue is the symptom of his "emotional sit-down strike."

From his study of hundreds of patients, Dr. Portis was able to pinpoint the causes and consequences of the flat sugar-tolerance curve. The vicious circle begins with poor eating habits—particularly, the absence of a good breakfast. This initiates the starvation of the brain, which alters brain physiology. The process now alters the impact of emotional stimuli on the body, and this in turn changes carbohydrate metabolism still more; and finally, the escape mechanism—the "emotional sit-down strike"—comes into play, as if the patient and his body had said in chorus: "If I can not have the gratification or activity upon which I insist, I refuse to make any effort." It is a rebellion against monotony and tedium and unwanted and disliked tasks that give no sense of achievement. A lack of zest, then, leads to a lack of sugar for the brain; and constant physical and emotional fatigue result, giving the jaded and disgusted an acceptable excuse for doing a poor job or escaping its responsibilities.

A psychiatrist, surveying this process, put it technically: "A condition of emotional letdown, based upon the disruption of the patient's goal structure, influences the vegetative balance and manifests itself in a disturbance of the regulatory mechanism controlling the sugar concentration of the blood. This produces the asthenic symptomatology and, particularly, fatigue. The fatigue favors the patient's tendencies toward withdrawal, impairs his efficiency, and discourages new effort." The practitioner, recognizing that treatment of the flat sugar-tolerance curve must precede, or at least accompany, any needed psychological treatment, then concluded: "In many cases, the somatic [physical] treatment is useful in breaking up this vicious circle, thus allowing a psychotherapeutic attack on the basic emotional problem." *

When the professional men intensely study the problems created by hypoglycemia and the flat sugar-tolerance curve—particularly the latter—they all become aware of the viciousness of the circle to which Dr. Alexander referred, where lack of zest deprives the body of stimulation needed to keep in tone the nervous systems that regulate the chemistry of sugar in the body. This leads to lack of sugar, which in turn creates zestlessness compounded by fatigue. Note that it is *zestlessness*, not *restlessness*. The person with the flat curve surrenders to fatigue because he is tired of it all. The other types of hypoglycemics will struggle against their fatigue.

Those who recall A. T. Cannon's concept of the "wisdom of the body" will remember that activities in which we participate with enthusiasm "tune up" the body in ways physiologically similar to those of fear and rage. So it is that one finds mild activity without emotional participation to be infinitely more tiring than strenuous activities into which you put "heart and soul." (Are dispassionate psychiatrists prone to fatigue?) If one is forced to participate in disliked activities—a job, for example, not even satisfying as a means to an economic end—the flat sugar-tolerance curve is created, resulting in chronic fatigue that

* Franz Alexander, MD, "Psychosomatic Medicine," *Proceedings of the Psychotherapy Council*, Vol. 2 (January 1944), pp. 41–60.

becomes pernicious and the climate for *all* activities, even those normally enjoyable.

It must be made plain that the root of the trouble is not merely an emotional reaction to lack of enthusiasm, to boredom, or to zestlessness. The fatigue and apathy that accompany activities in which one takes no interest are based on failure of the sugar-controlling mechanisms of the body to adapt to the effort required. The failure can be rectified with proper diet and vitamin supplements, but the basic cause will not be removed, obviously, and the fatigue will return if the emotional disturbance is not identified and psychologically treated. The curve can be normalized if the patient agrees to follow the menus I supply and take the vitamins I offer; but only the subject himself can come to grips with the problem of lost enthusiasm and attenuated interest in what he is doing. It is at this point that the patient will need psychological help, which physical improvement will aid. On this point, Portis remarks: "The rapidity of improvement of patients placed upon this therapeutic regimen [diet, medication] was striking. The small group of patients psychiatrically controlled showed an improved psychological status and a definite reduction of the period in which psychotherapy was needed. By this regimen the psychiatrist can be aided by the patient's more normal metabolism and his task made definitely easier." [*]

Portis states that he was impressed by the results achieved when treatment for the flat sugar-tolerance curve was combined with psychiatric therapy. The happy outcome was that the patient was able to lead a more nearly normal existence, with improvement in his emotional state, with increased efficiency, and with a return of zest and enthusiasm. He considers this approach to be useful for semi-invalids, who, because of the flat and featureless lives they lead, obviously run the risk of developing a flat sugar-tolerance curve. In elderly patients, the problem must be frequent, too, for there is no challenge in being placed on the shelf, but age obviously does not interfere with the response to Portis' treatment, for he finds it necessary to warn that elderly persons put on the hypoglycemia diet may feel so buoyant that they will overdo

[*] Sydney A. Portis, MD, "Life Situations, Emotions, and Hyperinsulinism," *Journal of the American Medical Association*, Vol. 142 (1950), pp. 1281–1286.

it if they are not warned that this treatment is not a fountain of youth. They can easily put too much strain on aged muscles and the circulatory system.

Let us now use this beam of scientific light to see who are the candidates for the kind of inescapable fatigue that comes from a flat sugar-tolerance curve, the physical expression of an emotional sit-down strike. Remember that this is the end point of monotonous, tedious, repetitive, unrewarding duties from which one cannot escape and which offer no challenge and no sense of achievement. Would not such a description fit the daily activities of many housewives? How about the bookkeeper, the cashier, the pieceworker, the car washer, the man wielding the wrench on the assembly line, the household domestic? If Thoreau correctly described most men as leading lives of quiet desperation, to what extent is the flatness of the sugar-tolerance curve part of the equation that sets the desperation quotient?

Certain studies have shown a particular vulnerability to hypoglycemia (and, particularly, to the flat sugar-tolerance curve) in a group of young business executives and their wives. The men's prestige and responsibilities in the business world would seem to insulate them against being jaded and zestless; the position, responsibilities, and economic advantages enjoyed by their wives would argue that they, too, would be immune. These views are superficial, and deeper probing shows that the young executive is often a victim of a business philosophy that will not allow him to stand still; i.e., he must be promoted or be fired. As he sees it, he gives the illusion of perpetual and high-powered motion, but he resembles the racing animal on the squirrel cage wheel—forever striving to gain, forever standing still. His wife, eager to escape the monotony of the endless pursuit of the Joneses, unable to meet with lesser figures in her feminine world for fear of violating the elaborate protocol of hierarchy that surrounds her husband, unable to escape from the monotonies of household duties, the children, her forever-tired husband, the evenings with TV because he is too exhausted to leave the house, the weekly bridge game, the PTA . . . she, too, becomes a victim of the flat curve, and the two sink into the gray fog of ubiquitous fatigue, too tired to enjoy each other or the children, too apathetic even to find catharsis in a satisfying fight with each other.

The diagnostic question is: are you tired or are you tired of what you are doing? If you can't answer, perhaps your physician and a six-hour glucose-tolerance test will.

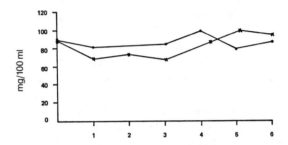

Here are examples of the "flat sugar-tolerance curve." This is a modified form of low blood sugar. The blood content doesn't drop after administration of sugar, but it doesn't rise to normal heights, either. The "flat curve" sometimes is the product of tedium, monotony; dull repetitive chores without a sense of achievement—and with no possible escape. Young executives who feel trapped will show this type of curve—and complain of fatigue, loss of zest, and boredom.

# 3. Prevent Hypoglycemia and Prevent Asthma, Hayfever, Food Allergies, Coronary Thrombosis, Epileptiform Seizures, Psychomotor Attacks, Peptic Ulcer, Rheumatic Fever, and ? ? ?

## Asthma

"The accepted forms of medical treatment for asthma among children are failing to cure the condition." So the newspapers quoted Dr. Vincent J. Fontana, director of pediatrics and pediatric allergy at St. Vincent's Hospital, New York City.

What are the "accepted forms" of medical treatment for asthma? Here is the story of a little boy who, by great good fortune, escaped from them. His history is typical of the experience of a large majority of asthma sufferers—typical, although only to the point where he encountered a practitioner courageous enough to leave behind the tried-and-untrue methods in favor of something experimental,* with the result that his asthma and virtually all other allergic symptoms disappeared. The boy was born into an allergic family, his genes threatening him with predisposition to asthma, hayfever, angioneurotic edema (giant hives), frequent colds, bronchitis, and eczema. Despite the roster of ancestral troubles he dragged into the world with him, in his first four years of life his only symptom of possible allergy was a series of tonsil infections, several of which were so severe that the swelling of the tonsils nearly closed off his air space. It became necessary to take a

---

* The weight of the consensus in medicine is formidable. It salutes a practitioner who uses the "accepted form" of treatment even if this treatment does little or nothing for a patient; it condemns and may even punish a physician who uses an "unaccepted form" of treatment, even if that treatment may help a patient. There is even a motto perpetuating this philosophy: Be not the first by whom the new are tried nor yet the last to lay the old aside!

calculated risk and remove the tonsils, for continued streptococcus infections—particularly in an allergic child—mean the possibility of rheumatic fever, although surgery on allergic tissue carries with it the risk of asthma, for it is known that trauma of any kind increases the reactivity of such tissue. Yet the doctor and the family really had no choice, for the boy was often in danger of asphyxiation from the severe and frequent tonsilitis. Surgery was inescapable. * Asthma followed a year later, after the child had been exposed to a heavy concentration of pollen, and his terrified parents, for the first time, but not the last, heard the boy gasp: "It takes all my strength to breathe."

Dr. Fontana's criticism of the "accepted forms of medical treatment for asthma among children" was justified when they were applied by all the many practitioners to whom the parents resorted. The boy's multiple allergies to food were identified, and the offenders removed from his diet. This proved to be something less than a mixed blessing, for the restrictions did not reduce the number or the severity of his attacks, but they did debilitate him—the taboo on all milk products, for instance, deprived the child of the calcium he needed for his growing bones. Moreover, calcium supplements could not be employed, for he proved allergic to these, too. In addition, his food allergies changed abruptly and without warning, and foods considered safe could suddenly trigger an asthma attack. His sensitivity to pollen and dust was identified, but this, too, was not rewarding. He was given a series of injections of these substances, beginning with the usual very low dosage, and progressing to greater concentrations, but his sensitivity was so exquisite that the allergist was never able to increase the dose to the point that would create a useful degree of immunity. In addition, each injection was likely to cause a cold, which would then be followed by attacks of bronchitis and asthma.

The family medicine chest reflected the futility of the whole regimen: it was jammed with potent but palliative medications to stave off asphyxiation, and these ranged from inhalants to aminophylline sup-

---

* As the reader progresses through this case history, he will learn that low blood sugar was the key to this child's problems. Apropos of his enlarged tonsils and adenoids, considered in the context of hypoglycemia, is it not interesting that there is a theory which indicts a high sugar intake in pregnancy as responsible for a baby's tendency to enlarged tonsils and adenoids?

positories and liquids, from antihistamines to corticosteroid hormones, each remedy presenting the risk of side effects almost as great a threat as the asthma itself. The overriding fear was status asthmaticus, which translates as asthma running riot, responding to no medication, and ultimately becoming lethal.*

Both parents became expert in administering adrenalin intramuscularly, by injection, a last-resort emergency procedure suggested by physicians weary of panic calls in the small hours of the night. The child became an example of retardation of growth because of restriction of the diet, possibly coupled with the poor utilization of certain nutrients, a phenomenon characteristic in severe food allergies. (Interestingly, some allergists have insisted that allergic children are *constitutionally* smaller than normal children, a thesis that ignores the acceleration in growth which may follow the restoration of a full and balanced diet.) An exposure to the wrong food, to a draft, to pollen or dust was enough to start the sequence in the little boy—from cold to bronchitis to asthma, occasionally varied by cold to sore throat to asthma.

From the always useful vantage point of hindsight, the child did show some symptoms strongly suggesting low blood sugar. He carried his lunch to school, like other children of his age, but unlike them, he also carried a snack to sustain him on the bus getting there. He was constantly and ravenously hungry, particularly for starches and sugars, and grew pale and irritable if he could not immediately satisfy his craving. He had an inordinate desire for salt, which he used in great

* There is a curious parallel between the asthmatic who becomes nonresponsive to the medications that once were palliative and the diabetic who has become "fast" or "brittle"—no longer manageable with insulin, even though dosage is high. In the case of the diabetic, I. M. Somogyi places the blame on overdoses of insulin because they bring a counterreaction in overproduction of adrenal hormones which the body uses to try to restore sugar levels in the blood. Frequently the medical approach to this problem is another increase in insulin dosage, which the body promptly checkmates again. Frequent medical approach to the asthmatic grown resistant to medication: higher and more frequent dosage of the same medications, some patients being driven to the extremity of injections of adrenalin every three hours! One is moved to conjecture upon the complexity of the scientific training needed to defeat the wisdom of the body.

quantities, a symptom of possible adrenal failure, which was also ignored. (Ineffective adrenals, permitting abnormal salt excretion, encourage large salt consumption. In the opinion of some practitioners —J. W. Tintera, for one, who has frequently published on this subject—inefficiency of the adrenal glands is a necessary prelude both to hypoglycemia and to allergy.) But the symptoms of low blood sugar in the child were never considered, paling as they did before the life-threatening attacks of asthma; and parents and child lived in a constant state of anxiety.

All the measures, the "accepted forms" of prevention and treatment of attacks—change of climate, electro-static cleaning of dust and pollen from the household air (expensive, but air conditioner filters are simply not adequate, the advertising notwithstanding), desensitizing injections, and medication—had failed. What next? A child psychologist—if the parents had not rebelled, for if ever a little boy had had an enlightened, loving, and yet not overprotective environment, this boy had. His mother, in fact, did consult a psychiatrist, just to be sure that in her anxiety concerning the child's asthma, she had not been shielding him excessively.

The parents themselves finally insisted on an investigation of their son's craving for salt and for sweets. They refused to be frustrated by medical blindness to hypoglycemia and its consequences and were determined to ascertain if these symptoms were in any way related to his problem. They persisted although they were flatly assured that the cravings were meaningless, that a high sugar intake is good for an asthmatic, that low blood sugar was not present (though a test had not been done), that if it were present, it would still have no relationship to asthma, and that hypoglycemia, if present, could easily be treated by feeding the child still more jam, jelly, candy, soft drinks, and sugar. Fortunately, instead of being overwhelmed by this parade of medical dogma based on solid ignorance, they continued to search until they encountered a medical nutritionist who was interested in the possible relationship between low blood sugar and asthma. He performed a six-hour glucose-tolerance test, which confirmed the presence of severe hypoglycemia. He also enlightened the parents concerning the folly of treating this condition with sugar.

Six months later, after strict adherence to the hypoglycemia diet, the parents realized that the boy had come through two severe colds without, for the first time, having them bring on asthma attacks, and from that point, they watched with increasing joy as his sensitivities to foods, pollen, dust, and bacteria faded. * In the six years that followed, his tendency to upper respiratory infection virtually disappeared, he had no asthma attacks at all, and he emerged with but one remaining sensitivity—an allergy to one type of seafood.

One child breathing freely does not make a case for hypoglycemia as a cause of asthma, but there are many other asthmatics who have responded positively to the diet, and there is a great deal of theoretical evidence to link low blood sugar with this and other types of allergic symptoms, some of which shall be outlined. It has been mentioned that fear of rheumatic fever was one reason for the surgery which was the prelude to asthma in the child. Is it not interesting that diabetics, whose blood sugar is high, of course, seldom show signs of rheumatic fever and therefore seldom have rheumatic heart disease, which is frequently the aftermath of rheumatic fever when it goes untreated? Abrahamson has reported, on this point, that rheumatic fever patients treated with the diet for hypoglycemia have gone through several winters without a flare-up of their disease, although many of them did have the type of streptococcus infection that ordinarily ushers in attacks of rheumatic fever. As he sees it, the evidence points to hypoglycemia as a factor in rheumatic fever: infection superimposed on allergic susceptibility, with low blood sugar—a by-product of a poor diet high in sugar and processed starches—pulling the trigger.

## Allergy

In discussing hypoglycemia in relationship to allergy, we must come to grips with the realization that the two conditions face a certain lack of

* The hypoglycemia diet for an allergic person, naturally, will be free of those foods that are irritants. However, as the person's condition improves and sensitivity decreases, forbidden foods (allergically speaking) can be restored to the diet in small, then gradually increasing amounts. See Appendix II, pps. 234 to 245, for a discussion of allergy testing, including methods which can be used at home; and the technique for spacing the intake of foods to minimize the risk of allergic reaction.

medical respect. As there are practitioners—too many—who do not recognize the incidence and the menace of hypoglycemia, so are there medical men who regard allergy as a "thing of the mind," cavalierly to be brushed aside. I still remember a resident physician who wished to administer a medication to which the recipient was violently and dangerously allergic and who refused to be deterred until the patient threatened to leave the hospital in his pajamas, if necessary, to escape the threat.

Elsewhere in this text the impacts of allergy are discussed, but those who recognize this phenomenon are far outnumbered by those blind to it and by those who reverse the equation and consider all allergy to be a product of neurotic conflict. Let us see, therefore, before we view the role of hypoglycemia in allergy, what explanation the allergist gives for such sensitivities and what they do to the sufferer, and then, finally, how hypoglycemia, as an unrecognized causative factor, contributes to allergy.

Let us say you react with an itch when exposed to sunshine or certain perfumes. You sneeze and your eyes water in the presence of dust. You have frequent colds, unrelated to epidemics. Pollen leaves you with a stuffed nose. You wheeze after eating eggs, get migraine headaches after eating chocolate, milk gives you a postnasal drip, insomnia follows corn, diarrhea follows coffee, or your hearing dulls or even disappears after you drink tomato juice. These and other common signs of allergy place you among fifty million Americans who suffer from this condition, that of "individuality gone berserk." The phrase is justified, for others can without penalty inhale, touch, and eat that which may put you to bed. You're lucky if your symptoms let you function, for some 14 percent of allergic people are seriously handicapped by their disorder.

Just as a diagnosis of a physical disease like an ulcer does not exonerate the patient from an accusation that this is an expression of a deepseated subconscious and unresolved conflict, so the diagnosis of allergy often invites a probe of the emotions. If you have an allergy, you are likely to be told that the affliction is—at least at times and at least in part—psychosomatic. You will be reminded that the asthmatic obviously needs to get something off his chest, that people itch when situations get under their skins, that there are events they cannot stomach, and that some intimates can be real headaches. So it is, you are told, that the complaints of the organs, coming at the end of a process called allergy, may really reflect emotional storms.

But let us assume that before you go to a psychiatrist to disinter your conflicts and, hopefully, resolve them, you are that most precious of rarities, a well-balanced person. Yet you are allergic. Why? You will be told that the disorder is the expression of your intense individuality, in which you react in a bizarre way to substances that to other people are innocuous. Since this is description, rather than explanation, it is analogous to "curing" your backache by tagging it as lumbago, a procedure that is often curiously semi-therapeutic but which in this instance leaves you dissatisfied.

Why does individuality go amok? When you press the allergist for a genuine explanation, he launches into a stage-by-stage description of the phenomenon, and once again you will be left with only one question: why am I allergic? He tells you that your body reacts to a food as it is supposed to react to the foreign protein of bacteria, or, for that matter, of organ transplants. The end product of this response is antibodies. These are responsible for the rejection of a transplanted organ and for your immunities against bacteria—which explains why the effort to avoid rejection of a transplant by depression of this protective mechanism often condemns the patient to severe, and sometimes fatal, infections or cancer. (History may forgive our ignorance. Will it condone our pretensions?)

In the case of a food, an antibody reaction can cause nothing but trouble, for food, unlike a bacterial invasion, is a frequent visitor to the body, and the production of antibodies can and does reach abnormal levels. At some point, the surplus antibodies begin to attach themselves to the cells, instead of circulating freely, and when fresh antigenic material comes in contact with the cell-attached antibodies, an explosive reaction takes place, in the course of which cells are destroyed. The disrupted cell material causes the release of histamine, a chemical which in excessive amounts is responsible for much of the reaction you suffer when you eat the offending food; hence the antihistamine pills, which, since they intervene in the process at a late stage, do not cure but do palliate the symptoms of allergy.

One of the effects of histamine is an increase in the permeability of cell walls, which, in the case of blood vessels, allows blood serum to go into the surrounding tissues, where it does not belong, and the result is inflammation and swelling of the areas. Hence the water-logged nose, the hives, the itching, the asthmatic chest, the tearing eyes, and all the other distressing symptoms that make allergy so difficult to bear.

This is a dramatic portrayal of a biochemical war within the body, but it still does not tell you how and why the war started. If you press the point, the beleaguered allergist will finally resort to informing you that (a) the tendency is universal, for allergy is simply a perversion of the normal immunizing mechanism of the body, and (b) that the tendency is obviously genetic, for allergies do tend to run in families. These slightly contradictory statements do have one virtue: they relieve the psychiatrist of the burden of explaining what unresolved conflicts preceded the entrance into the world of a baby born with an allergic eczema. They also again beg the question of why others can eat, touch, inhale with impunity that which immobilizes you.

The theory that charges hypoglycemia with some of the responsibility for provoking allergies at least gives us a foothold on a basic premise. For the first time, we have the opportunity to interrupt the series of biochemical reactions that end in allergic symptoms, not at the stage where trouble looms, but long before. The theory is not esoteric, involves no secret remedies, and is fortified by the best possible combination of types of evidence—experimental (animal research) and clinical (trial on allergic human beings). Like so many other promising findings, this was presented in a paper now gathering dust in the medical libraries. It was among those delivered at a meeting of the Federation of American Societies for Experimental Biology, reported in the *Journal of the American Medical Association*, May 18, 1963. The title given to it by the medical group is as myopic in its way as the group's philosophy on public health: "A New View of the Old Cold—as Sugars Go Up, Hypersensitivity Drops." It is a nearsighted view of a finding that is applicable to the relief of the suffering of millions of allergic patients, although the paper itself does, more or less perfunctorily, point out that colds are frequently a manifestation of allergy and become more severe when blood sugar is low, a fact that supports the wisdom of the old folk advice to feed a cold! But this report discusses the role of low blood sugar in the common cold merely as a springboard toward a much more sweeping examination of the relationship between hypoglycemia and severe allergic reactions, for it cites experiments on animals that demonstrate that all allergic reactions are worsened by low blood sugar, and some—the lethal type—will not occur at all if sugar levels are normal. The author demonstrates that it does not matter by what means the blood sugar is lowered—insulin, oral drugs of the type used to treat diabetes, or starvation. When hypoglycemia has been established, the test animal, challenged with an allergy-producing substance, responds with a life-threatening allergic reaction.

The researcher, Dr. Vincent Witold Adamkiewicz (PhD), has thereby for the first time given us a clue to *the* start, or *a* start, of the process that leads to allergy, and his findings represent important corroboration of the benefits that have accrued to asthmatics and sufferers from hayfever who, treated for concomitant hypoglycemia, responded by losing their allergies. Such cases are reported by a number of medical authors, Gyland and Salzer among them. Dr. Adamkiewicz' discovery removes the recovery of such patients from the area into which scoffing allergists place it: "spontaneous remission" or "delayed response to previous medication."

The theory still leaves much to be explained. We still, for instance, don't know how and why a decrease in blood sugar level triggers allergy, but at least we are rid of description masquerading as explanation, for we now have a clue to the process that triggers it all—that which precedes individuality gone berserk: it is a deficit in blood sugar. This leads to an interesting thought. If low blood sugar paves the way to allergy, should not diabetes, with its high blood sugar, protect against it? *

The proposition is not so logical as it may seem, for diabetics, after all, are sick people, and their elevated blood sugar is only part of their manifold biochemical aberrations, from which, perhaps, no dividend of any nature should be anticipated. Yet the theory is tempting—logical enough to have led me on a fruitless chase of nonexistent evidence, some years ago, when Sandler, a physician, proposed the concept that hypoglycemia is the necessary prelude to susceptibility to polio (and perhaps other virus infections). He showed that animals normally im-

---

* Let the reader remember that undoubtedly there are other causes and other contributions to allergy. We are dealing with a neglected factor.

mune to polio have relatively high levels of blood sugar, but lose their immunity when their blood sugar is lowered by injections of insulin. Sandler, who also believed that coronary attacks may be invited by low blood sugar, published his findings a few months before his home city— on the basis of prophecies of past experience with polio—anticipated a serious epidemic.

A newspaper reporter reviewed the Sandler book, and frightened mothers, reading that cola and other sweetened drinks, candy, ice cream, cakes and cookies, and excessive intake of sugar might make their children more susceptible to polio, suppressed their children's cravings for sweets. There were two results: the sale of sweets fell to an all-time low, and so did the incidence of polio that summer. This could have been coincidence, but it did relate logically to Sandler's experiences of trying to induce polio in animals with normal blood sugar. The development of the Salk vaccine, of course, slammed the door on this avenue of approach to the polio problem, though it might have led us to more basic and better weapons against other viruses, against which we still have no vaccines. Parenthetically, the incident does lead to an interesting, if disturbing thought: if excessive sugar intake, leading to an oversensitized pancreas, overproduction of insulin, and consequent low blood sugar, make our children and us more prone to virus infection, what service is performed by fluoridation, which, in the words of Dr. Frederick J. Stare, of the food-industry-subsidized Harvard nutrition department, "allows the children to go on eating their sticky sweets"?

Dr. Sandler's theory raised other urgent questions, such as whether or not diabetic children are susceptible to polio. They are known to be more resistant to colds, but this has been ascribed to their diets being better balanced than those of normal children. Did their excess blood sugar protect them? And did it help them to avoid polio? The polio foundation was queried for data, but although this agency claimed that it followed up all clues, however improbable or unpromising, it replied no information was available.

Allergists who were queried agreed that diabetics are less likely to be allergic, and the incidence of diabetes in the allergic population is far below the incidence in the general public, but one practitioner said he did have a patient—just one—who was both diabetic and allergic, and insisted that it took only one to explode our "beautiful theory," as he put it. With his cooperation, a six-hour glucose-tolerance test was made of this patient, and the "beautiful theory" survivèd, for the results showed the presence of both diabetes and hypoglycemia. This, the reader will recall, is called "dysinsulinism"—the pancreas being under-active in the first few hours after the administration of sugar and then going from diabetic underactivity to the overactivity that yields low blood sugar. This, of course, would indeed make it possible for a diabetic to have periods of possible allergic reaction.

Now scientific interest took me to the opposite investigation. If sugar-tolerance tests were made routinely on a random sample of asthmatics, what percentage of them would reveal hypoglycemia? Such a group was tested. Twenty-five percent of them were clearly hypoglycemic. More would have been so labeled had it not been for the shortcomings of the test method and the standards of appraisal of normal blood sugar, for the test used lasted two hours—the typical test for diabetes, which will not reveal dysinsulinism—and the patient who showed "only" a 10 milligrams percent drop below fasting level at the second hour was considered normal. The reader here should remember that Gyland labeled such patients as pre-hypoglycemic. Treatment of hypoglycemia in such patients did cure their asthma! Had the longer test been performed and Gyland's standards employed for its evaluation, I do not doubt that the result would have been what both Gyland and Abrahamson found: hypoglycemia in virtually all asthmatics.

There are, of course, many other "coincidences" that tend to relate hypoglycemia to asthma. I do not think, for example, that it is pure chance that all the hormonal materials used to treat asthma share at least one action: they all raise blood sugar. This is true of adrenalin, of cortisone, and of other such drugs. It is also true of all the so-called sympathomimetic medications, drugs which simulate the action of the sympathetic nervous system. Many of these are used to relieve not only asthma, but also many other allergic disorders.

One would suppose that allergists would be interested in the observation that drugs which raise blood sugar dominate the list of those which help the asthmatic. Several allergists did in fact subject many asthmatics to glucose-tolerance tests, but they were looking for diabetes, did not find it, pronounced the patients in this respect to be more normal than nonallergic people, and terminated the investigation. The test they employed was a two-hour glucose-tolerance test, which, as the reader now knows, may completely miss the type of hypoglycemia that is most common—that which reveals itself only in the later hours of a six-hour test. Another factor inimical to the allergists' recognition of hypoglycemia as a factor in allergy is the question of the standards by which they would judge low blood sugar. Many of Gyland's patients—including the asthmatics who were cured—were not hypoglycemic when measured by the textbook.

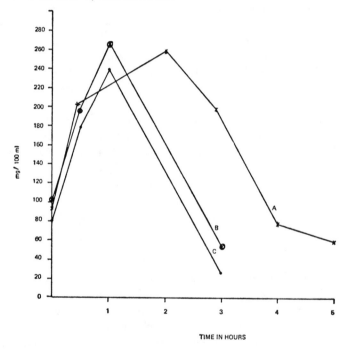

TIME IN HOURS

A five-hour test for low blood sugar reveals the danger of stopping at the three-hour mark. Note Curve A, which is diagnostic of low blood sugar in the four- and five-hour tests but deceptive at the three-hour mark.

There are diametrically opposed differences between asthmatics and diabetics. It has often been observed that the two diseases seem mutually exclusive: an asthmatic who develops diabetes loses his asthma. In

families where the tendency toward both diseases seems to be transmit-
ted genetically, it is extremely rare that both appear in one individual.
Another difference appears in the effect of thyroid hormone, doses of
which are helpful to asthmatics and harmful to diabetics. An overactive (toxic) thyroid will gravely worsen diabetes. It has also been no-
ticed that asthmatics tend to concentrate potassium in the blood, while
diabetics show rather low blood serum potassium. Excessive salt harms
the asthmatic, but large amounts of salt have been found to reduce the
insulin requirement of diabetics, though the treatment, which necessi-
tates a tube into the intestine, is not really a practical one.

It is interesting that injections of glucose (sugar) are sometimes used
to stop severe attacks of asthma.* If such injections *cured* the patient,
the theory of low blood sugar from hyperinsulinism would seem to be
invalid, for temporary rises in blood sugar would of course touch off the
pancreas, with a resulting overproduction of insulin which would drop
the blood sugar, thereby allowing the patient to secure only temporary
benefit. Actually, that *is* what happens; injected glucose (and the large
doses of sugar by mouth that have been recommended for asthmatic
children) give but fleeting benefit, after which another asthmatic attack begins. Conversely, the type of diet formerly used to treat epilepsy
has been employed with success in treating asthma. This is a high-fat,
high-protein diet, quite low in carbohydrates—which is, of course, a
description of one of the diets for hypoglycemia, and the coincidence
has meaning, both for asthma and for certain types of epilepsy.

* The tendency of asthmatics to have attacks in the small hours of the night
and early morning would of course suggest that hypoglycemia is involved. It is
strange that this observation has never received the attention it deserves, if
only because of the coincidence that in the same hours, gastric ulcer trouble
tends to attack—at the time when, dinner long since digested, blood sugar
tends to sink to a low. If pollen is regarded as the chief trigger for a given case of
asthma, why should the attacks occur at the time of the night when the pollen
count is apt to be lowest? If emotions alone are the trigger for gastric ulcer
attacks, why do they tend to strike at the hour when sleep is deepest and the
level of emotional stress presumably the lowest? And while I am on the subject—with reference to Sandler's indictment of hypoglycemia as contributing
to attacks of coronary thrombosis—is it coincidence that many of these heart
attacks occur also in the small hours of the night, when snow-shoveling,
emotional stress, and exercise cannot possibly be factors?

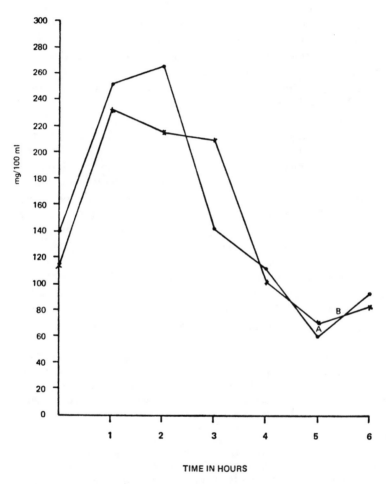

TIME IN HOURS

High fasting levels of blood sugar are no guarantee that low blood sugar is not the cause of the person's troubles. Note here the high initial values, suggesting a diabetic tendency, followed by drops of 72 milligrams percent below fasting level in Case A and 44 milligrams percent in Case B.

Before discussing the epilepsies, a few added notes on allergy are needed. Though the discussion to this point has been concerned with asthma, there is evidence that low blood sugar may play a role in hayfever, too, as well as in other types of allergic reactions. It should not be thought that the hypoglycemia diet is the only weapon among nutritional armaments that is useful in allergy. From what has been said about the effect of histamine on the permeability of cell walls, it is obvious that any nutrient that inhibits the action of histamine should be helpful. Vitamin C has such an effect because it destroys histamine and is destroyed by it. This explains two phenomena: the tendency of allergic individuals, whatever their diets, to have low blood levels of Vitamin C; and the antihistamine effect that Vitamin C dosage creates in many allergic people. A rise in Vitamin C levels in the blood, far beyond the amount needed merely to avoid scurvy, will make an active antihistamine carrier of the blood and should simultaneously help to reduce the permeability of the cells, which increases in Vitamin C deficiency and during excess histamine activity.

Elevated histamine levels are not confined to the blood of allergic individuals. There can also be high levels of histamine in the tissues. In addition to its role in allergies, such tissue histamine may be responsible for depression. Along with Vitamin C, therefore, I use calcium and methionine, which over a period of time—maybe as much as six months—will lower the tissue histamine levels. Antihistamine drugs, incidentally, will not do this; their action is confined to histamine in the blood. Calcium and the bioflavonoids have similarly desirable effects in normalizing the permeability of the cell walls. These observations bring a perspective on the vicious circle that the allergy diet, often severely restrictive, may bring into being, for allergy to citrus fruits and milk products, sources of the helpful factors we have been discussing, often makes their presence in the diet impossible, yet deficiency in their nutrients intensifies the symptoms of allergy. Nutrient supplements can be helpful for those not allergic to the concentrates themselves. There is no way to predict the reaction to the supplements, for allergy to citrus fruit does not necessarily mean allergy to Vitamin C or the bioflavonoids; nor is allergy to calcium necessarily present with an allergy to milk. The cooperation of the medical man is the sine qua non, because he is needed for the glucose-tolerance test, prescription of the hypoglycemia diet, and recommendation of needed supplements. Thus it is most unfortunate that many medical men, hampered by medical tradition, will choose to ignore the possibility of hypoglycemia, or deny its etiological role in allergy. And it is equally unfortunate that they will not properly control the hypoglycemia diet, if they do prescribe it, but will allow or even encourage the intake of sugar, and will prescribe supplements, if at all, with an attitude of "they won't do any good, but they won't hurt you."

These deficits in medical competence in recognizing and managing hypoglycemia—whether alone or complicated by allergies—present the layman with a problem which to an expert is a challenge. It is frequently very difficult to reconcile the dual set of dietary prohibitions with which an allergic hypoglycemic must struggle. Some foods that are permitted in the hypoglycemia diet may be taboo because the patient is allergic to them. Sometimes, in multiple allergies, choices become so limited that the patient is literally unable to make choices of foods for his menus. On pages 198 to 210, you will find that I have assembled the information available to help in coping with both problems.

The physician who does not have a high index of suspicion for hypoglycemia, or who considers it to be a rare disorder, is not likely to test the hypoglycemic for allergies resulting from or contributing to the low blood sugar. Visiting a conventional allergist may not yield any dividends for the hypoglycemic with allergies. It may astonish you, but orthodox allergists are not yet convinced that food allergy is as prevalent as I know it to be, and an even larger majority vigorously deny that there is any such thing as allergy affecting the brain. In part, this negative attitude derives from their definition of allergy. If a food does not produce a rise in the blood level of Immunoglobulin E, then you are not allergic. This negative attitude holds even though after eating the food, you feel weak, listless, depersonalized, spaced out, or highly irritable. The situation with allergies in hypoglycemics closely parallels that with allergies in arthritics. Despite the fact that it has been irrefutably established that allergies can trigger or worsen arthritis, my experience is that one arthritic in five hundred has been investigated for allergies. To give you some help in identifying the presence of allergy, I am going to outline a number of tests for allergy, some of which must be administered by the physician, some of which you can do yourself.

In extremely aggravated allergic conditions, fasting for a few days in an environment from which nonfood allergens are excluded—meaning that the air must be pure, as well as the water, for I have seen hypoglycemics whose allergies were worsened by constant exposure to water containing chlorine, fluoride, or both—may be the only fruitful resource, but it is my strong conviction that this must be done under medical supervision. There are clinics for in-patients, in several parts of the United States, where such medically supervised fasting is administered. Fasting would be dangerous for those with active cancer, advanced diabetes, or tuberculosis, as well as for pregnant women, women who have just given birth, and children who, obviously, need constant nourishment to support growth.

In case you decide to ignore my cautions and fast without medical supervision, it is not only necessary to go into a fast gradually, but to be cautious when you reintroduce foods. If you mix them, you will not know which one caused symptoms. Some of the mixing may be inadvertent—like an anonymous sauce on a vegetable, creating symptoms blamed on the vegetable, but actually caused by one of the ingredients in the sauce. Your reaction to a fried egg may not be an egg sensitivity, but allergy to the fat in which it was fried. After you have abstained from food, an allergic reaction may not appear the first time that you eat one of the real offenders. The body tends to recover its balance when you abstain from a food to which you are allergic. That is the reasoning behind rotation diets, which introduce four-or five-day delays in repetition of favorite foods. In fact, there is an axiom: it is the foods you love the most that are most likely to be the offenders, because you have eaten them often enough to touch off the allergy mechanism. In essence, after a fast, you are deliberately testing foods. This may be done without fasting, by the simple process of elimination of suspicious foods. There is, though, a possible trap in this process. For example, you may think that you are allergic to wheat, but eliminating bread or wheat products produces no change in your symptoms of allergy. The easy conclusion is likely to be fallacious: you may actually be allergic to wheat, but the allergy is mild and does not trouble you until simultaneously you take a second food to which you are also allergic. Allergies can be additive.

If you want to try testing by elimination of foods that you suspect, you should eliminate all of them if possible, or at least as many as you can. You begin by removing from your diet the foods you crave. Logic will often dictate that the first foods to be eliminated are milk, wheat, corn, chocolate, and eggs, because these are frequent offenders. They should be eliminated from the diet for a ten-day period before testing. During those ten days, be careful to confine yourself to foods that in the past you ate infrequently. They are less likely to be sources of trouble.

Basic foods can be ingredients in other foods that you may not consider as possible offenders. Needless to say, bread is not the only source of wheat. Many of our convenience foods contain numerous ingredients, and you may be eating foods you wish to eliminate when you don't suspect it. This means that *you must read labels*. Also, few laymen realize that there is cross sensitivity among foods. For example, if you are sensitive to tomato, which is a member of the nightshade family, then other members of that family would be suspect. In Chapter 10 you will find a list of food families for your guidance.

It is paradoxical but true that symptoms of allergy may grow worse during the first few days of withdrawal from offending foods. Be of good cheer, for that situation reverses. If you don't have either of these responses, and your symptoms go on unchecked, food allergy may not be your problem, or the foods that you are putting to the test are not offenders for you, or, as sometimes happens, this type of testing is not your cup of tea and you must resort to some other method. On the other hand, marked improvement or complete disappearance of the symptoms invites the introduction of the eliminated foods, but one at a time. Do not anticipate an immediate allergic reaction if the food that has been reintroduced is in fact allergenic for you. It may take a few days of eating each of the foods you return to your diet to determine whether it is an offender or innocuous for you. If restoring a food reawakens symptoms, obviously you should discontinue it, and stop testing until the symptoms subside. There is one safe conclusion: if removing a food from your diet brings an improvement in your symptoms, and returning to that food ignites the symptoms again, you have performed an allergy test as valid as any that might be conducted by an expert.

I have left one bit of bad news for the last. Smokers must stop smoking during the period when suspect foods are being removed from the diet, for sensitivity to tobacco is frequent, and, indeed, allergic addiction may be the basis for addiction to cigarettes.

## The Epilepsies

Epilepsy, until recently, was considered somehow shameful—the disease was such a stigma that one gathers that the afflicted would rather plead guilty to positive Wassermann tests than acknowledge epilepsy! Most people know, rather vaguely, that there is more than one type of epilepsy; some know that many gifted people have had the disease; practically everyone imagines that all epileptics are subject to convulsions. Actually, the convulsive type (grand mal) differs sharply from the others. There is petit mal, in which the seizure may merely be a blinking of the eyelids, an instant of blankness, after which the sufferer returns to normalcy, such attacks coming once or twenty times a week, or twenty times a day, or even more frequently, so that life to him is somewhat like a motion picture in which a frame, visual or auditory, here and there, has been cut out. There is psychomotor epilepsy; there is a traumatic type, following physical injury to the brain; there is the group called epileptiform, where the disease may be expressed as gastric cramps, migraine headache, or in some other form in no way resembling the classical concept of epilepsy; there is the jacksonian type, and there are still many others.

I am here addressing the psychomotor type, though it is entirely possible that in selected cases my discussion may apply to other types of epilepsy—petit mal in particular. The evidence that invites research into the relationship between low blood sugar and psychomotor epilepsy and petit mal is found in a number of interrelated clues:

1. Many adolescent—and some adult—epileptics show a distinct craving for sweets. It is entirely possible that in some of these cases of sweet tooth, hypoglycemia is present and acting as a trigger for attacks.

The relation between time of attacks and the spacing of meals, the consumption of sweets and cola beverages, and the time of day of the attack itself (night or day) may offer clues to the presence of low blood sugar, but the absence of such evidence still does not preclude the possibility that a six-hour glucose-tolerance test may confirm the presence of hypoglycemia. If hypoglycemia *is* present, treatment must be undertaken, for if it does not initiate epileptic attacks, it may worsen them.

2. The electroencephalograms (tracings of electrical brain waves) in petit mal are curiously like those in hypoglycemia.

3. Psychomotor epileptic attacks are known to be triggered by factors of stress, which may be emotional, glandular, allergic, or arising from hypoglycemia. There are cases where soft drinks containing both caffeine and sugar have been known to trigger attacks within twenty minutes after consumption.

4. The type of diet found most helpful to epileptics is "ketogenic." This diet produces a mild type of "acidosis"—which is placed in quotation marks to distinguish it from the type of indigestion that the public similarly labels. This acidosis is believed to anesthetize the nerve endings, thereby protecting against attacks. A ketogenic diet is one in which the ratio of carbohydrate to fat is much lower than in the everyday diet. This, of course, is also a description of the diet for hypoglycemia, excepting that in the latter the fat-carbohydrate ratio is adjusted so that the ketogenic effect does not occur or is mild and transient.

Another clue is found in an interesting report by a physician who, forced to play medical detective, discovered the cause of the Monday morning attacks that had become routine in a group of children whose epilepsy had otherwise been perfectly controlled through a ketogenic diet. He had determined for himself that sugar and caffeine were both undesirable for his patients, on the empirical basis that attacks were fewer when colas, sweetened or unsweetened, coffee, and tea were deleted from the diet. He finally realized that the Monday morning attacks followed Sunday trips to the movies or amusement parks. It took little deduction to indict the cola drinks, candy, ice cream, and popcorn the children had consumed when not under the strict dietetic supervision exercised at home. The doctor's comment did not mention hypoglycemia, though it squarely placed an accusing finger on the types of foods and beverages known to aggravate low blood sugar.

I have seen hypoglycemics who had been assured that they had aberrant types of grand mal since they had the blackouts but not the typical "spike waves" in the encephalograms. I have known children with psychomotor epilepsy whose troubles flared within a half hour (or less) after consumption of a cola beverage and whose symptoms closely paralleled those of hypoglycemia (though not investigated on that basis): increasing paleness, obvious anxiety, irritability, maniacal outbursts of rage, weakness, and then, finally, the psychomotor attack. Readers fortunate enough not to be acquainted with this condition should note that it is sometimes misconstrued as sheer and malicious delinquency. These patients will rip drapes and curtains off the wall, slash furniture, set fire to inflammable household materials, trip a passing adult, with no discernible provocation assault another child—and then be completely dazed when punished by their parents, behaving as if they had no consciousness of what they had done and no comprehension of the sudden punishment.

Many physicians, whose suspicion of hypoglycemia is seldom aroused, will balk at a six-hour glucose-tolerance test for a child. Yet an epileptic—at any age—is entitled to such a test, or, failing this, to the therapeutic diagnosis of a trial of the diet itself. When small children are involved, caution must be exercised in the use of ketogenic diets, which require strict supervision, for the carbohydrate-fat ratio that produces but a mild and harmless acidosis in one child may in another of the same age yield it in an undesirable degree. This caution, however, does not bar use of the diet for young children, but merely urges competent supervision; for older children and adults, of course, the hypoglycemia diet presents no such problems.

There are, of course, epilepsies of a number of types that do not involve hypoglycemia or allergy. I have for many years researched nutritional therapies in brain damage of some. In cases deriving from deprivation of oxygen via cardiac arrest, or damage to the brain from inhalation of carbon monoxide, or physical trauma, I have employed a nutritional therapy which on occasion has been remarkably effective in restoring consciousness and at least some degree of cognitive function in patients whose original prognosis was "chronic vegetative state." In the course of that clinical research, it was inevitable that I would encounter patients who developed epilepsy as one of the complications of their brain injury. In a significant percentage of these cases, nutritional therapies were effective in reducing the frequency, duration, and intensity of the epileptic attacks. Accordingly, I applied the treatment in a number of these cases of epilepsy of unknown origin. In a percentage of these cases, it stopped or reduced the frequency of the attacks. The therapy involved the use of octocosanol, which is a long chain waxy alcohol derived from wheat, accompanied there by hexacosanol, triacontinol, and tetracosanol. Carnitine, a protein normal to the body, which aids in the metabolism of such fatty acids, was employed with the octocosanol. Copper, which has powerful anti-inflammatory and anticonvulsive effects, was also used, as well as taurine (an amino acid). There have been patients who were hypoglycemic and had epileptic seizures, for whom this therapy increased the effectiveness of the hypoglycemia diet in controlling or, in some cases, eliminating the convulsions.

## Gastric Ulcer: Wound Stripe of Civilization?

One need not be a nutritionist to recognize the marked similarities between the diet for peptic ulcer and that for low blood sugar: there is the same emphasis on frequent, small meals; the same prohibition of coffee, tea, and cola beverages; the same taboo on concentrated sugar; the same emphasis on fat and protein.

The parallels go beyond this. One British author (T. L. Cleave) makes a strong indictment of sugar as a principal cause of gastric ulcer. The painful cramps of hypoglycemia and the pain caused by gastric ulcer are so strikingly similar that X-ray studies have been performed on hypoglycemics in a vain search for stomach ulcer. I have already pointed out another similarity: the empty stomach is a hazard in both disorders, explaining why peptic ulcer attacks so often come at two or three o'clock in the morning, the hours at which hypoglycemics tend to awaken and then have difficulty in returning to sleep.

These similarities largely have gone unnoticed, not only because hypoglycemia has interested only a handful of medical men, but because the psychiatrists have put the entire responsibility for peptic ulcer on the emotions—pure nonsense, for nutritionists have demonstrated several types of mild dietary deficiencies that will cause spontaneous ulcers in animals. This concentration on emotional factors has allowed the gastroenterologist to ignore the possibility that low blood sugar, which can cause gastric distress indistinguishable from that caused by ulcers, may be responsible for these "wound stripes of civilization." While civilization does bring its tensions with it, it also doles out, let us remember, over one hundred pounds of sugar per person per year!

It is known that there are relationships between body structures and constitutional susceptibilities to certain diseases. Students of morphological characteristics have pointed out that gallbladder sufferers and diabetics share many characteristics of structure, but gastric ulcer patients are constituted quite differently. In any case, it is of interest that diabetics tend to escape stomach ulcer, and when they do have both diseases, glucose-tolerance tests have sometimes shown the familiar pattern of dysinsulinism. However, this is not the only reason for considering low blood sugar as being conducive to gastric ulcer. There have been studies made of patients with stomach ulcer in which the six-hour glucose-tolerance test was given and the hypoglycemia diet prescribed. *All* the patients showed hypoglycemia, and *all* showed beneficial response to the diet, many of them completely escaping the frequent doses of alkalies that ordinarily are given to ulcer patients.

If you mention the preceding information to your favorite psychiatrist, he will point out that his services are needed along with the prescribed hypoglycemia diet, for hypoglycemia itself is a stress-produced disorder. Or, conversely, he may insist that the stress of having gastric ulcer may be enough to cause hypoglycemia! To him—and to others who have overstated the case for the emotions as the *sole* pathway to gastric ulcer—I pass Abrahamson's observation that the troops in combat in World War II had fewer ulcers than those in the training camps. He points out that the trainees had easier access to sugar and to caffeine-containing beverages. They're scarce on the battlefield, although emotional stress isn't.

# 4. Low Blood Sugar—an Organ Recital

The human pancreas manages to be two different kinds of glands simultaneously. One of them produces digestive secretions that reach the intestine via two ducts to help in the utilization of all forms of food—fat, protein, and carbohydrates. The other is an endocrine (ductless) gland that, as the name implies, releases a hormone directly into the blood circulating through that part of the pancreas. The hormone is well known to diabetics; it is insulin, a protein substance that has two functions in which we are vitally interested: it helps us to burn sugar, and it aids in recycling our reserve sugar supplies when they are needed by the body.

Because insulin is a protein substance, diabetics, who need supplementary supplies of the hormone, must take it by injection, for—like any other protein substance—when it is taken by mouth it is promptly digested, losing its identity and function as a hormone.

The pancreas, which may be between six and eight inches in length, runs along the rear of the abdominal cavity, its right end connected with the small intestine. This arrangement enables the digestive secretions of the gland to aid in the digestion of food. Its left end is in the neighborhood of the spleen, a placement that has no purpose. Overactivity of the pancreas produces many symptoms, which are discussed in this book, but only one physical symptom that the physician can detect at will, in a physical examination. That sign is a tenderness at the point in the abdominal area related to the position the pancreas occupies. Perhaps it is not coincidence that a similar sensitivity appears in children deficient in Vitamin B Complex (a group of vitamins that have many functions in the utilization of sugar) in the same general area as the pancreas is located. Such a sign of vitamin deficiency may be apparent in children who by all other standards are "well fed."

The pancreas fails to control blood sugar in diabetes. This failure, the tendency to which may be genetic, may rest upon inadequate production of insulin, or it may derive from a counterreaction by the body, in which insulin-blocking substances are produced in excessive amounts. There may also be a blockage at the insulin receptors at the cells. Physicians attempt to cope with this situation by prescribing dosages of insulin (or oral blood-sugar-lowering drugs) and by controlled diet.

The medical man gauges the effectiveness of these controls by checking the amounts of sugar in blood and urine. Actually, this is a workaday accommodation to an oversimplified view of diabetes, for as every medical man and every nutritionist knows, the disease involves more than high blood sugar, more than a shortage of insulin or an oversupply of its antagonist. The biochemical disturbances go far beyond a difficulty in proper utilization or recycling of carbohydrates. Diabetics, for instance, do not share with healthy people the process by which the body derives a substantial part of its Vitamin A supply. They are unable to convert the vitamin precursor (carotene), present in fruits and vegetables, into the true Vitamin A. They may improperly utilize fats and have difficulty, for example, managing cholesterol. Their biochemical management of proteins appears to be disturbed, as well as their utilization of at least one mineral. And though there is primary attention given to the functioning of the diabetic's pancreas, autopsies have shown that this gland will sometimes appear to be normal, with a normal or even a high content of insulin, while the diabetic's liver will show evidence of disturbances in function and even alteration in structure.

All these considerations are to us incidental, for this book is concerned with the opposite of diabetes—not with high blood sugar, but low. Since low blood sugar (hypoglycemia) can have a number of causes, the medical term used to describe the cause that interests us is "hyperinsulinism"—overproduction of insulin. We can refine that definition still more, for we are not interested in hyperinsulinism that results from a tumor of the pancreas, and arrive finally at idiopathic, functional hypoglycemia: low blood sugar that does not have an organic cause (such as a pancreatic tumor). "Idiopathic," however, is misleading, for it means that the cause of the disorder is not known, the medical dictionary defining such a condition as "self-originating" or "of unknown origin." Actually, I suspect that the most common cause of so-called idiopathic, functional hypoglycemia is hyperinsulinism caused by excessive intake of sugar and caffeine and compounded by emotional stress. *

The role of stress in altering blood sugar levels—up or down—comes as no surprise. Physicians treating Wall Street brokers have long said that they need not look at stock prices in the newspapers; they can gauge what is happening by the amount of sugar excreted by diabetic brokers. Similarly, army physicians observed during World War II that the stress of aerial combat frequently gave pilots a transient diabetes. The emotional links between the thalamic brain and the pituitary gland, the relationships among the pituitary, the adrenal glands, and the pancreas are more than just recently recognized.

Not only does the pituitary manufacture a hormone that raises blood sugar and pushes the body in the direction of diabetes, but the body has still other mechanisms to offset the action of insulin in lowering blood sugar. This balancing process in part depends on the adrenal glands, which under stress will nudge the liver into releasing stored sugar (glycogen) so that there is fuel available for fight or flight. Those same adrenal hormones, in the absence of any stress, will still begin activity if the blood sugar level falls, as it does when insulin is released. Thus we have a picture of a balancing mechanism that is dynamic, prepared to compensate for any deviation of blood sugar from the level needed to keep brain and nervous system (which depend on sugar for function and, indeed, survival) properly nourished. This emphasis on adrenal hormones should not be construed as endorsement of the thesis, long urged upon the public by some lay "experts" in hypoglycemia, that every patient needs injections of adrenal cortex hormones. In my experience, covering thousands of patients with low blood sugar, about 90 percent of them have an adrenal deficiency which is not direct but relative to overactivity of the pancreas. This is to say that in such patients when the pancreas is quieted, no longer stimulated by sugars, the adrenal has the capacity to return to normal functioning. In 10 percent of the patients, there is a direct failure of the adrenal glands.

* This is a deliberately oversimplified view of possible causes of functional low blood sugar. Liver function is probably involved; so may be deficiency in an anti-insulin hormone, glucagon. Likewise, enzyme chemistries play a role.

These are the patients who profit by injections of adrenal cortex. The discussion is academic, since the United States Food and Drug Administration, with its monopoly on scientific knowledge, has decided that adrenal cortex should be removed from the market, on the grounds that it does not contain enough cortisone to be useful. Its cortisone content, however, has nothing to do with its medical use, and one can only hope that the government will overcome its lag. There are perhaps twenty-five hormone principals in adrenal cortex, other than cortisone, and there is no doubt that the benefits patients receive from this treatment do not derive from the cortisone content. In the supplements I use in treating hypoglycemia, where I suspect that the adrenal is not performing its task of raising blood sugar, I often employ supplements of pantothenic acid and para-aminobenzoic acid (paba) to stimulate adrenal function. For some patients it is quite effective.

So it is that the body is prepared to counter *sudden* deviations from the normal level of about two teaspoonfuls of sugar in the bloodstream. What it cannot tolerate is *continued* deviation—whether in the form of consistently overelevated blood sugar levels—or, what is even more threatening, consistently depressed blood sugar levels. The body can long endure elevated blood sugar, but the opposite condition proves intolerable. Moreover, medical tests quickly identify elevated blood sugar but may miss the opposite condition for reasons this book fully explains.

The explanation of the system by which the body protects the blood against too much and too little sugar in the blood begins with the way in which food is converted into energy. As you eat and digest a meal, the breakdown products of the food are passed to the blood which goes to the liver—not to that which goes into circulation around the entire body. Were this not the arrangement, two slices of bread would so jam the blood with sugar that each of us, at least immediately after a meal, would be diabetic.

In the liver, the sugar—now in the form of glucose—is converted into glycogen, which is the form in which the body can store sugar, since it is now no longer capable of being dissolved in water.

Insulin, like Vitamins B1, B2, and niacin, has been likened to the wick of a candle or an oil lamp: something that helps us to utilize the fuel at the rate we desire. But this hormone goes beyond that function; it is as if the wick had the power to turn the kerosene into a solid fuel, allowing us to store the reserve without worrying about evaporation. The analogous action of insulin on our sugar-fuel is to turn it from glucose into glycogen. If this were not the arrangement, the sugar in the blood, reaching the liver, would pass right through into the general circulation, swamping it; and in the liver no reserves would accumulate, to be drawn on to replenish blood supplies as a balance against the action of insulin.

Now we can trace the destination of that piece of bread, potato, or lump of sugar: it goes into the specialized circulation, reaching the liver in the form of glucose. None of it has been burned, up to that point, for there is no insulin present. When the sugar-carrying blood leaves the liver, the rise in the fuel content touches off the pancreas, which now releases insulin, the hormone passing directly into the blood. The insulin is now carried by the circulation back to the liver, where it works upon the sugar coming from the stomach and intestines and converts it into the insoluble glycogen, for storage. The removal of much of the sugar from the blood now leaves the amount the body needs, which the insulin now helps each cell to burn properly.

The process is all neatly balanced, and the puzzlement is not that it so often goes wrong, but that it remains normal in so many of us. Just speculate now on what happens if the amount of insulin produced is out of proportion to the amount of sugar reaching the blood and the liver! Consider that the resulting drop in blood sugar would in turn stimulate the adrenal glands into activity. The adrenal hormones have an action opposite that of insulin: they raise blood sugar, but they do that, it must be remembered, by forcing the conversion of the stored sugar (glycogen), which does not dissolve, into ordinary sugar, which does. This release of the adrenal hormones, whether or not the pancreas is overactive, is also responsible for the internal feelings of alarm (anxiety) that plague so many victims of hyperinsulinism. It is also the cause of the "idiopathic postprandial syndrome" (see page 245).

The liver does not have a monopoly on the ability to change glucose into glycogen, or back again, nor on the ability to store the insoluble form of sugar. It is shared by the muscles, though the task is largely dominated by the liver.

This partial and schematic tour behind the anatomical and bio-chemical scenes is included so that the reader may appreciate the delicacy with which this system is balanced and the formidable troubles that may start with a slight imbalance in any segment of the sequence. Complex as it is, this system may be compared with an automobile tire, which performs its function efficiently and in silence as long as it is in balance. But just affix a one-ounce weight at any point on the rim and watch the intense vibration that now develops and threatens to wrench the tire away from the wheel! Let me make a further analogy: consider the carburetor of an automobile engine to be roughly equivalent to the insulin mechanism of the body, and the fuel to be equivalent to the sugar in our food. If the carburetor is set at too rich a mixture (analo-gous to high blood sugar), the engine falters, runs roughly, and stalls. If the mixture is too lean (low blood sugar), the engine has difficulty in starting, may overheat, and stalling again results.

The adjustment on a carburetor is a simple one—reducing or in-creasing the amount of fuel reaching the engine. The parallel adjust-ment when the body's fuel is being burned too fast is really just as simple—a revision of the diet. It seems too simple, which explains why the opposite condition, diabetes (too much fuel), has virtually monop-olized medical and lay attention. Diabetes has within it an essential drama—a successful medical battle against a gene-controlled disease that used to be a definite death sentence but is now reasonably well managed through insulin injections, oral drugs, diet, and nutrient ther-apy. There are no dramatic treatments for hypoglycemia—just a diet, control of allergies, and a vitamin supplement. The response is neither quick nor immediately dramatic, though ultimately it represents just as great a triumph as control of diabetes. Perhaps it is more of a triumph, for untreated diabetes ultimately brings symptoms that are clearly rec-ognizable indications of physical disease, whereas neglected hypo-glycemia simply lets the patient sink into a cotton-swathed gray morass in which he is neither truly sick nor truly well and doesn't know why!

Hypoglycemics outnumber hyperglycemics: there are probably at least two people suffering from low blood sugar for every one afflicted with diabetes. Moreover, every physician, from bitter experience in giving this hormone to diabetics, is familiar with the appalling con-sequences of overdose of insulin. The existence of "upside-down diabetes"—hypoglycemia—was recognized many decades ago, just two years after F. G. Banting identified insulin. Yet, with all this, hypoglycemia remains a stepchild, ignored by medicine, unknown to the public. One cynic has suggested that a "wonder drug" is needed for hypoglycemia, some kind of miracle remedy that can be packaged and labeled with glowing promises of quick relief from the fatigue, anxiety, insomnia, irritability, and unprovoked weeping caused by low blood sugar. That would popularize the disease with the public. Instead, the diagnosis of low blood sugar takes effort, time, and money, and the treatment demands that the very foods craved by the patient—sweets, cookies, pies, cakes, candy, soft drinks, coffee, cola beverages—be avoided. Sometimes tobacco, too, is prohibited. No public relations man in his right mind would try to popularize such a disorder!

To return to the history of the recognition of low blood sugar, the first hint was obtained in 1924, after insulin had been in general use for about a year. Physicians had learned to use the drug with great caution, having watched diabetics go into shock from slight overdoses of the hormone, and the medical journals were filled with observations and cautions from medical men who had become aware that this great boon to diabetics had to be used with competence, discretion, and awareness of its two-edged properties. Dr. Seale Harris, professor of medicine at the University of Alabama, made an important observation: there were people who were not taking insulin—people who didn't have diabetes—who appeared, nonetheless, to be suffering episodes of insulin shock. Like every medical man, Dr. Harris was aware that endocrine glands are all capable of being overactive, and he investigated the possibility that the pancreas in some people could produce excessive amounts of insulin. This he found to be true, and so reported in 1924.

Other medical men added their contributions, making clearer the existence of hyperinsulinism and identifying the causes—for there proved to be more than one. Tumors of the pancreas, benign or malignant, can, if located in the insulin-producing area, be responsible for overproduction of the hormone. These conditions, fortunately, are very rare. If the tumor is not malignant—which in this area would often mean death—surgery readily cures the condition. However, operations are the last rather than the first resort, even for the nonmalignant pancreatic tumor, for this condition is often brought under excellent control by the hypoglycemia diet.

A third cause of hyperinsulinism, also responsive to surgical treatment, is an enlargement of the entire insulin-producing area of the pancreas (the islets of Langerhans), the enlargement being generalized, meaning that there is no lump or tumor.

The fourth cause for excessive production of insulin, the one with which this book is concerned, is purely functional. There is no cancer, no tumor, no general enlargement of the insulin-producing tissue. The pancreas has simply been oversensitized to sugar and is overactive in producing insulin or underactive in producing glucagon, the hormone that is anti-insulin in its effect. This is the response to too much prodding of the organ by the brain and the nervous system and to too much tension and anxiety, producing an imbalance of nervous impulses reaching the pancreas or a collateral disturbance of the function of the liver in meting out its stores of reserve sugar. This is the price paid for eating over one hundred pounds of sugar a year and for drinking the bottomless American cup of coffee, lavishly sweetened, alternated with innumerable bottles of caffeine-containing beverages, similarly oversweetened. The combination of caffeine and sugar is particularly unfortunate, for while the sugar is stimulating the pancreas into activity, the caffeine is attacking by another route—the adrenal glands. These, the reader recalls, have the capacity to induce the liver to convert its glycogen back into sugar, which, of course, goes into the bloodstream, combining with the sugar that sweetened the coffee. To the pancreas, the source of the sugar makes no difference: it will produce insulin whether the sweet is coming from the sugar bowl, a bottle of pop, or the reserves stored in the liver. The latter organ is a vital part of the mechanism that controls our blood sugar. S. Soskin has shown that dogs with the pancreas removed, fed large amounts of sugar, will—if *normal* amounts of insulin are supplied—maintain normal blood sugar. One would expect that the absence of increased insulin production to meet this challenge would result in a diabetic curve, but the liver manages to control and stabilize the blood sugar level, nonetheless. This authority on carbohydrate metabolism has shown that dogs with liver function disturbed, pancreas removed, and normal amounts of insulin supplied are *not* able to control blood sugar levels, which then mount to diabetic heights.

These observations, which illuminate the importance of the liver in control of blood sugar, bring into focus an action of the sugar and of other highly processed carbohydrates in the American diet. These fractionated sugars and starches have so been processed that factors important to liver function have been depleted or removed. Therefore, it may be that the mischief worked by such foods for the hypoglycemic is in part from overstimulation of the pancreas, but also partially from the insult to the liver caused by vitamin deficiencies that inhibit its control of sugar reserves. Such vitamin deficiencies would also affect the utilization of sugar within the cells, including, of course, those of the nervous system and brain, thereby adding to the impact of hypoglycemia on these systems. This technical note is given so that the reader will understand why the hypoglycemia diet included in this book is supplemented with Vitamin B Complex concentrates. Despite the propaganda campaigns calculated to persuade us that we are the healthiest and best-fed people in the world, there are many times when a supplementary supply of vitamins becomes critical. This is so when it is a question of hypoglycemia that is the result of a dietary history of excessive intake of sugar and other vitamin-poor carbohydrates. *

From the previous discussion of the action of caffeine, it is obvious that unsweetened coffee via adrenal control of reserve sugar in the liver can stimulate the pancreas into activity. This phenomenon makes the black coffee so beloved of dieters a poor choice, for its temporary effect of depressing appetite is really based on its action of pushing reserve sugar into the bloodstream, an action that also provides the temporary lift. This obviously is unfortunate for hypoglycemics (many of whom are overweight), for the process must ultimately lead both to challenging the pancreas and the adrenals, causing low blood sugar, and to the increased appetite that makes dieting that much more difficult. Coffee is bad not only for those with hypoglycemia, but for anyone who uses it

---

* It is fashionable today to regard vitamin users as faddists. Soskin, no faddist but an internationally known specialist in carbohydrate metabolism, suggests that *all* of us need a Vitamin B Complex supplement because of our consumption of overprocessed carbohydrate foods.

as a "pickup," for the lift is only temporary, and is earned at a physiological price.

Anyone who has truly suffered the penalties of low blood sugar is usually willing to eliminate candy, sugar, heavily sweetened foods, and the caffeine-bearing beverages from his diet. If the symptoms are persuasive enough, the patients will without complaint drop liquor and tobacco, too, and the coffee and Danish pastry breaks, and the canned fruits packed in heavy syrups, * as well as the cereals pre-sweetened by the manufacturer. Such action, of course, will bring attention to the patients, for society feels itself threatened by those whose behavior strays outside the accepted norms, and this is true, too, of nutrition and health care. Anyone who makes an effort to eat to meet physiological needs—whether in the treatment of hypoglycemia or its prevention, as an example—is obviously some kind of crackpot, for only a health nut tries to stay healthy.

These are the very real pressures on the hypoglycemic and those who would rather not be. The norms of the menus in America are painstakingly defined: only a faddist will eat an apple and a bit of cheese as a dessert when one can be "normal" and gulp down apple pie à la mode, with 18 teaspoonfuls of sugar per portion! If you drink freshly squeezed vegetable juice, you are philosophically akin to a little old lady in tennis shoes; but if you drink canned vegetable juice that has been heated, blended, and homogenized, you are a loyal, normal American. You put yourself outside the pale of dietetic respectability when you quench your thirst with pure water. Why should you when you can instigate or aggravate hypoglycemia (and erode your teeth) by choosing cola drinks that combine the acidity of vinegar with the pancreatic impact of 5 teaspoonfuls of sugar blended with a dollop of caffeine or sweetened with a questionable protein?

The mention of pure water brings up an important point. There are many individuals, not necessarily suffering from low blood sugar, who

---

* The amount of sugar that reaches us from syrup-packed fruits is unbelievable: sugar-packed canned pears yield 80 calories per cupful, while water-packed ones (without added sugar) yield only 36. Sugar-packed apricots supply 110 calories per cupful; water-packed, only 45. The difference lies solely in the added sugar. Juice-packed fruits simply supply sugar from a different source.

cannot tolerate the chlorine and the fluorides in most drinking water supplies. In addition to that, there is solid evidence that hard water confers many health benefits, including increased resistance to cardiovascular disease. Investment in a good mineral water is rewarded: mineral water supplies several factors, including calcium and magnesium, in which the hypoglycemic's previous diet has frequently been deficient.

So, if you prefer "normal" health, read no more. If, on the other hand, you're willing to run the risk of genuine well-being, plus being ostracized by your debilitated peers, read on. I am about to describe the process by which physiological needs in diet can be combined with pleasures of the palate, for the two are not necessarily mutually exclusive, which is to say that the degenerated taste buds of the average American can be reeducated to find pleasure in foods that are good for him.

The first step is to reduce the intake of sugar and overprocessed carbohydrates of all types.

A medical nutritionist at the University of Alabama medical school remarked that people "give themselves little sugar-tolerance tests every morning." He was talking about the "quick energy" breakfasts that produce nothing but fatigue for millions of hypoglycemic Americans, some of whom obviously flunk the tests. This medical man, who has shown that less than a week of abstention from the highly processed sugars and starches can significantly tighten loose teeth in "healthy, well-fed subjects," was not exaggerating. The breakfast of orange juice, Danish pastry (or muffin or doughnut), and sweetened coffee yields an intake of processed carbohydrate that is startling—large enough, certainly, to challenge the pancreas as the physician deliberately does when he insults the islets of Langerhans with a dose of 100 grams (3⅓ ounces) of sugar.

A glass of fresh orange juice normally yields about 20 grams of sugar, and the sweetened variety supplies about 26 grams, so that the eye-opening glass of cold juice has one 25 percent of the way toward the full-scale sugar-tolerance test. (It should be noted here that there appears to be some difference in the impact of the unprocessed sugars, as they appear naturally in food, and that of commercial white sugar on the hypoglycemic. This impression requires more investigation, for scientifically, it makes no sense, yet the medical nutritionist previously quoted has the same impression concerning the impact of unprocessed versus processed carbohydrates on the stability of the structures that help retain the teeth.)

A Danish pastry contains about 17 grams of quickly absorbed, over-processed carbohydrate, and if one is not satisfied with that, there are always the varieties filled with jam (55 percent sugar, 45 percent fruit). A jelly doughnut yields about 30 grams, roughly an ounce or 8 tea-spoonfuls of sugar. A chocolate milk, choice of teenagers and inaliena-ble "right" of small American children, yields over 31 grams plus a stimulant analogous to caffeine. Since the caffeine in coffee causes sugar to be released from the liver, we must speculate on the amount, but we can count the 2 to 4 teaspoonfuls of sugar with which millions of Americans sweeten each cup of their favorite breakfast beverage. The cola drinks, likewise, produce the caffeine effect and the known con-tent of 20 grams of sugar in a six-ounce glass. The sugarless varieties still elicit discharge of sugar reserves through the action of caffeine.

Now, total the intake of sugar and highly processed starch from such foods and beverages, from such breakfasts and snacks, and you can get an idea of how near average Americans are to eating their way into a full-scale sugar-tolerance test before the day is half over.

Perhaps, as Abrahamson noted, it is not coincidence that the symp-toms of hyperinsulinism were first noted at the University of Alabama's medical school, for in the heat of the South, many natives will con-sume three, four, five, or even six bottles of a cola beverage between breakfast and lunch! If reduction of so preposterous an intake of sugar, which is a condiment rather than a food, is not justified by the risk of initiating or aggravating hypoglycemia, consider that sugar intake has been linked to many disorders that in the public's understanding are not even connected with diet. Gastric ulcer and hemorrhoids and periodontoclasia (weakening of the structures holding the teeth) are among these. Sugar has also been charged with responsibility for arte-riosclerosis and heart attacks, which the public blames on cholesterol.

It is not enough, though, merely to reduce sugar intake. It is desir-able (a) not to overeat of carbohydrates and (b) to change the form in which carbohydrates are taken. There are significant nutritional dif-ferences between whole wheat bread and white bread, for example, and this is universally true of most whole grains as compared with the commercial, highly processed equivalents, which were devised originally, if you have forgotten, because of the need for stable, cheap foods that could be warehoused without the risk of rodent and weevil infestation. This objective was achieved by the creation of food that will not support life, food that the lower animals and insects would avoid.

Thus brown rice is a better nutritional choice than white rice, converted rice being a compromise between the two. Whole corn meal not only tastes better but is nutritionally superior to the commercial degerminated product. One should remember here that foods which keep should neither be kept nor eaten, for when they are so highly processed that even oxygen avoids them, man should be similarly wary.

Whole rye is better nutritionally than commercial rye flour, which is analogous to overprocessed white wheat flour. Thus commercial rye bread offers no nutritional advantage over what foreigners call our "bubble gum," plastic commercial white bread. How could it? It is made from 45 percent overprocessed rye flour, blended with 55 percent overprocessed wheat flour. *

Contrary to popular belief, other than honey, there is no commercial form of sugar that is a contribution to good nutrition, and about honey, there are still some questions to be asked, for much of its sweetness comes from the same glucose we are trying to avoid. Brown sugar is just white sugar contaminated by a bit of molasses, and raw sugar offers no benefit significant enough to justify its price. Blackstrap molasses does not deserve the eulogies given it by the nutritionally incompetent, but it is a much richer source of calcium and iron than dark molasses, which in turn is much richer in calcium and iron than the light molasses. Guess which the public, with its instinct for the mediocre in foods, prefers!

So it is that choosing carbohydrate foods in the nutritionally better, unfractionated form is as important as controlling the percentage of

---

* Pumpernickel is equivalent to the commercial rye bread, fermented and given an artificial suntan with burned sugar. The term "caramel color" on the label indicates this. Genuine pumpernickel—whole rye grain bread, fermented— requires no cosmetic treatment. Commercial whole wheat bread is generally a good buy among packaged products.

calories from such foods in the diet. Do you find any logic in stuffing yourself with sugar and these refined sugars and starches until you develop constipation which then has to be treated with the bran and bulkage previously removed from these foods? Is it to you poetic justice that you consume the overprocessed breakfast cereals and then buy what was removed from them as "nutritional improver" for your diet?

University students, pondering those considerations, will usually ask: "How much bread should I eat? How much cereal? What percentage of the diet should be starch and sugar?" Such questions are asked in terms of the healthy person's needs and must so be answered. The hypoglycemic requires much more stringent restriction of sugar and starch intake, as does the pre-hypoglycemic. The person who is not equipped to handle carbohydrates efficiently—whether or not he is headed for hypoglycemia—and who is possibly identified as such by his family history of diabetes, his tendency to dental caries, or the ease with which he gains unwanted weight on carbohydrates may require a level of intake of sugars and starches below the average (50 percent of calories in the diet from such foods) and above the amount tolerated by hypoglycemics. These are the areas of individual differences that are anathema to the authorities, who must assume that we will all be equally well fed on the same menus, and frustrating to the layman, who would like precise directions in selecting his nutrition for good health—as long as they don't bar him from his favorite foods. Unfortunately, as long as our biochemical differences are greater than our similarities, it will be necessary for each of us to work out his own dietetic destiny. That truism will continue to be ignored, of course, by the "Establishment," which will go on pretending that "a good mixed diet" gives a guarantee of good nutrition to all. The situation closely parallels that in education, where we have long proceeded on the premise that all children are equally educable, thereby pretending that we have no need for special classes for slow learners, enriched curricula for fast learners, and sheltered environments for dullards.

We have now decided to reduce sugar intake, keep carbohydrates at 50 percent of the total calorie intake (or less, if the patient is hypoglycemic, diabetes-prone, overweight and resistant to ordinary reducing diets, or in some way evidencing the presence of the caveman's gene for efficient utilization of starches and sugars) and to select our carbohydrates largely from the unfractionated, unprocessed forms.

The effects of sugar on the body are quite different from those of the complex starches. Some complex starches act like simple sugars. See the glycemic index, page 217 to page 220. In a comparison of Boston Irish with their counterparts in Ireland, the European group showed a resistance to hardening of the arteries associated with heart disease, while the Boston group was quite susceptible—and the only difference of significance in their diets being the substitution of sugar in the American diet for the potatoes of the Irish menu. It would be sensible to reduce sugar intake, then, by at least 80 percent—to perhaps fifteen or twenty pounds a year. This reduces sugar from a major source of calories (more than 200,000 a year in the American's diet) to its original role: a condiment. One does not eat one hundred pounds of a condiment per year—not without ill consequence.

Eating highly processed carbohydrates entails many nutritional penalties. Do you find any logic, for instance, in arguing for or against the need for vitamin supplements when your patronage encourages manufacturers to continue removing Vitamin B6 and Vitamin E from cereals, flour, and other carbohydrate foods? Does it make any sense to you that the pacifarins that help to protect against infection are removed from wheat when it is processed into white flour? Shall we continue fruitlessly to dose infertile women with hormones (like dropping seeds into unfertilized soil, if nutrition is not improved, reported a Cedars of Lebanon Hospital research group) and condone the continued removal from our carbohydrate foods of pro-fertility factors like para-aminobenzoic acid? Lest you think that this information comes from an esoteric source, let the reader review the observations by Benjamin Sieve, MD, endocrinologist-nutritionist, who was able with simple doses of this one vitamin (paba) to restore fertility to 12 of 22 women, all of whom had been infertile for at least five years.

Many of the factors removed from the carbohydrates in processing are concentrated in the grain germ, from which comes new life when the seed is planted. This is removed because its high concentration of nutrients makes it susceptible to oxidation, which shortens shelf life. The processors have so deftly managed their propaganda that those who attempt to eat grains with the germ intact or who consume the germ itself (wheat germ, for example) are considered by the consensus of debilitated Americans to be food faddists. This social pressure should not discourage you from using wheat germ to restore nutrients to processed cereals, to white flour in baking, and to bread crumbs in appropriate dishes. Wheat germ is highly perishable and should be purchased only in vacuum-packaged containers. It should not be defatted. These days, it may be contaminated with EDB, a highly toxic insecticide.

Although American mothers have been persuaded that a breakfast of cereal and milk is basic nutrition for a school child, the fact is that many of these concoctions bear more resemblance to candy than to a cereal food, and, indeed, the criticism bears more examination, now that manufacturers are actually adding marshmallow to these "breakfast foods." A bowl of cereal may be good food if it is whole grain, but in simple terms of calories, it is but equivalent to a slice of bread, and not very good bread at that, when one considers the long processing and high temperatures to which many cereals are subjected in the roasting process. A visit to a dry cereal factory is a revealing and a shocking experience to those with any perspective on the impact of processing on nutritional values. There you can see the germ of the corn being carried away, destined for animal feed, for animals, having a cash value, are important, and must be given the benefit of the high protein, vitamin, mineral, and unsaturated fat value of the germ. The starch that remains is ground, flaked, and roasted, with an addition of the inevitable flavoring agents and sugar.

The removal of the entire Vitamin B Complex, minerals, protein values, and unsaturated fats is then "compensated" for by "enrichment," this being the restoration of one vitamin for every three removed. In many cereals, artificial flavor and color are added.

There is no validity in the distinction made between dry and cooked cereals, there being poor foods among both, but generally speaking, oatmeal remains a better buy, and all whole-grain cereals (preferably devoid of the additive BHT) are good nutrition. The cereals spiked with a half-dozen vitamins may bring some benefit to those whose vitamin nutrition is poor, though a properly balanced vitamin supplement would be preferable. In any case, breakfast should feature a protein food—eggs, meat, fish, fowl, or cheese—with cereal offered only if appetite is then not satisfied. Wheat germ added to a cereal will vastly improve its nutritional value, as mentioned previously, and is itself a fine breakfast cereal, with a protein value of fine quality and of a percentage exceeding that of meat.

The timing of American meals also requires modification. We do take between-meal snacks for the good reason that a pattern of three meals a day is a concession to timetables and has no relationship to physiological needs. What this book tells you about the blood sugar curve—its amplitude and frequency—should persuade you that more frequent refueling, with five or six small meals to replace three larger ones, makes more biochemical sense. Our snacks now tend largely to increase the sugar-starch intake, and the sensible rule is a simple one: in each of the five or six small daily meals, take a protein of animal origin—meat, fish, fowl, milk, cheese, or eggs. Because of what dietitians call the "complementary effect," these animal proteins, which are capable of supporting growth and maintenance of the adult structure, improve the efficiency of the inferior vegetable and cereal proteins when the two types are ingested simultaneously (or within an hour of each other). As an example: the protein of beans, not complete in all the protein factors the body needs for growth and maintenance, is complemented by the better protein of the frankfurter when the two are taken within an hour or less of each other, but that effect disappears if, for instance, the beans are taken at lunch and the meat at dinner. This complementary effect of proteins is of more than academic importance, not only because it is the most expensive type of food, but because a good part of our protein intake is in the form of the less complete and less efficient vegetable and cereal types. In terms of the low-income budget, for example, the household cook is displaying our most advanced nutritional knowledge when he or she makes oatmeal with nonfat milk powder, thereby boosting the value of the oat protein to that of the milk, while utilizing the least costly source of fine milk protein.

The amplitude and frequency of the rise and fall in the sugar levels, mentioned a few times back, refers to how high the sugar curve goes, how low it drops, in what period of time, and how often during the day. The medical man places much emphasis on the *fasting* level of blood sugar as the base line from which he derives much of his data and some of his conclusions. Actually, though, the fasting blood sugar level represents an abnormal state, a kind of starvation. Your fasting level may be 72 milligrams percent of blood sugar. Your *normal* state—that which will keep brain and nervous system fully functioning—will be nearer to 120 or 140. The object of more frequent meals is to help you to keep the blood sugar away from the physician's base line—the fasting level—and up toward the functioning level. If all this seems technical to you, let us hope that one day you have the opportunity to observe a kymograph machine that is recording the hand tremors of an individual who boasts that he needs only one or two real meals a day. Without breakfast, his tremor increases markedly, a visible sign of the dissatisfaction of his nervous system with his system of timing meals.

From all these data, there are conclusions that logically follow. It is obvious that those who skip breakfast present their bodies every morning with the challenge of functioning in partial famine. Those who adopt a pattern of frequent, small meals, on the contrary, are stabilizing the blood sugar levels, avoiding not only transient starvation, but sudden rises and sudden drops in blood sugar levels. This is most important, for it is the elevation of blood sugar, not the amount of the rise that touches off the pancreas. An increase from 80 to 120 miligrams percent of sugar in the blood will produce as much pancreatic activity as a rise from 180 to 220. Since, as part of our somewhat subversive effort to remain healthy, we are trying to avoid sensitizing this organ, it is obviously better to smooth away the jagged peaks in the blood sugar curves, representing large sudden rises.

Another dividend from the frequent meal pattern may be better control of blood cholesterol. There is evidence that man does better as a nibbling animal than as a ritual eater of the same amount of food in three large meals daily. Even though the food intake is the same in both instances, the rise in blood cholesterol is less when the meals are frequent and small—and the deposits of fat are fewer. This means that this pattern of eating also makes it easier to control weight or to reduce, not only because it helps to bring appetite under control, but because the body appears to be less efficient in utilizing a given amount of food divided into small rather than large meals.

Many medical writers on nutrition hesitate to recommend high-

protein diets, citing them as expensive. This displays the same ignorance of food economics that most people display, for the costliness of
protein is in large measure due to their shopping preferences and preju-
dices. Fish, less costly than meat and fully equivalent in protein content and value, is neglected by the American, who buys some thirty-
five pounds of it as against hundreds of pounds of meat. Meat itself is
purchased on the apparent premise that the entire animal is made up of
choice cuts—sirloin, T-bone, ribs, roasts, filet mignon—and the buyer
will thereby attempt to outbid his or her neighbor for this limited
assortment. The law of supply and demand operating here as it does
anywhere else, the prices of these preferred cuts soar while those of
hundreds of pounds of perfectly good meat from the same carcass—the
block chuck—will be lowered so that the butcher may recover his
investment. Of 125 cuts of meat on the market, the average buyer may
know of twenty and concentrate his or her buying on about a dozen. In
so doing, that person not only runs counter to the laws of economics,
but those of good nutrition. The healthy man is the whole man, and
the healthful food is the whole food, in this case, the whole animal.
Thus, meats should not be taken solely from the muscle cuts, which are
the popular ones, nor from the block chuck alone, but also from the
organs. In eating liver, sweetbreads, hearts, lungs, and kidneys, one is
consuming the whole animal, as primitive man did and does, right
down to the bones and their marrow, exactly as, in eating whole wheat
and brown rice, one is choosing the unfractionated, whole food. Remember that the word "healthy" means whole. A healthy man is a
whole man and helps himself to preserve physiological integrity and
buoyant well-being by eating the healthful, whole food. In the case of
meat, this doctrine will help the average buyer avoid trying to outbid
his or her neighbor for a handful of overpriced cuts, while the rest of
the animal, which is at least as palatable and often more nutritious,
remains in the butcher's showcase, awaiting a buyer too knowledgeable
or on too strict a budget to eat unintelligently.

Some of the foods mentioned in the preceding paragraph are among
the particularly rich sources of the Vitamin B Complex, a group of
vitamins I have already emphasized as being of particular importance to
those whose carbohydrate metabolism is disturbed—diabetics, for in-

stance, and, of course, hypoglycemics. Returning to the doctrine that what nutrition helps, it helps to avoid, it is obvious that anyone seeking to retain good health should favor liver function by a generous intake of these vitamin factors. Vitamin B Complex does not refer to the three B vitamins that are restored to enriched white bread. These are arbitrarily selected from a group that also includes (usually in the same unprocessed foods) pyridoxine (B6), folic acid, paba, pantothenic acid, inositol, choline, and a group of unknown factors (not yet identified, therefore not yet titled.) To remove nine vitamins from flour and restore three can be called enrichment only by the generous in spirit, and the deficit, which includes factors critical to liver function, the utilization of fats, and the functioning of nervous system and brain, is a disservice to the American consumer trying to preserve good health. Contempt of those so inclined has prevented all but health-food-store patrons from using, for instance, brewer's yeast, which is an extraordinarily concentrated source of the Vitamin B Complex, so much so that it has been used (originally on the basis of folklore) to help diabetics control their blood sugar. Carbohydrate processors prefer to label with derision such supplements as "health foods"; this is obviously a less costly ploy than the proper restoration to their products of the vitamins now removed and not returned.

Let us now review the recommendations:

1. Reduce the total intake of carbohydrates, with particular emphasis on sugar.

2. Take all carbohydrates, wherever possible, in the unfractionated, unprocessed, or less highly processed forms, with the consideration of the glycemic index (see p. 217).

3. The food intake that maintains proper weight should be divided among five or six smaller meals, rather than three large meals daily. Breakfast should be substantial.*

---

* These recommendations require some clarification. Although I find smaller, more frequent meals, each containing a small amount of animal protein, to be better for health and prevention of low blood sugar than the customary meal pattern of three large meals, the first meal of the day should nonetheless be substantial. The absence of breakfast, or relying on a juice-cereal or juice-muffin type of breakfast, is the first step toward hypoglycemia.

4. An animal protein should be included in each of the meals. Choose among fish, fowl, meat, milk, cheese, eggs.

5. In selecting meats, try to consume more of the total animal. Use organ meats as well as muscle cuts (steaks, chops, roasts). Liver, kidney, lung, heart are good foods.

6. One of the purposes in using organ meats is to increase your intake of the Vitamin B Complex. Fortify this intake by adding to your diet such concentrated sources of these vitamins as brewer's yeast and wheat germ. Brewer's yeast is available in forms that taste like meat and like cheese. It can also be used in tablet form. *

Americans, prideful in their land of plenty, assume that poor diet and inadequate medical care are the monopoly of other races and other ways of life. But no one consistently eats an ideal diet, nor would any one menu plan meet all the varied requirements of millions of people. Poverty and ignorance are not the only pathways to nutritional inadequacy. Consider, for instance, this chart of causes of vitamin deficiency, and then realize that it is incomplete:

FACTORS PREDISPOSING TO VITAMIN DEFICIENCY †

I. *Indequate Intake, owing to:*
   1. Poverty
   2. Ignorance, including improper preparation of food
   3. Working conditions
   4. Available foods
   5. Cultural patterns and faddism
   6. War-stricken areas
   7. Diet fads
   8. Gastro-intestinal disorders, such as anorexia, vomiting
   9. Chronic alcoholism
   10. Advanced age
   11. Prolonged intravenous glucose infusions

* The recommendation of the use of Vitamin B Complex supplement is in addition to the suggestions made in the sixth recommendation. Not only does Soskin recommend the use of such concentrates as a sensible prophylaxis for all who eat the overprocessed carbohydrates, and not only does Abrahamson use concentrates of all the vitamins—the B Complex included—for hypoglycemics, but I have noted the beneficial responses to vitamin supplementing exhibited by hypoglycemics and, indeed, thousands of other individuals, both sick and presumably well. When millions of Americans are counting calories, a calorie-free vitamin concentrate easily fits into the scheme of things dietetically, especially where high-vitamin foods may be rejected because they are high-calorie, or, if used, taken in quantities too small to be useful.

† *American Practitioner*, Vol. 13, No. 8 (August 1962), p. 19A.

12. Restricted diets in treatment of:
    a. Peptic ulcer
    b. Gallbladder disease
    c. Diabetes mellitus
    d. Colitis
    e. Allergy
    f. Obesity
    g. Convalescence
    h. Infant formulas not including orange juice or equivalent
13. Neuro-psychiatric disorders
14. Adentia
15. Pregnancy

II. *Impaired Absorption*
1. Gastro-intestinal disturbances
    a. Chronic diarrhea
    b. Chronic ulcerative colitis
    c. Coeliac disease
    d. Tuberculosis
    e. Absence of bile (obstructive jaundice)
    f. Surgical resection of considerable portion of intestinal tract; other surgical procedures, such as of pancreas.
    g. Achlorhydria or achylia gastrica
    h. Persistent vomiting, as in pregnancy, pyloric stenosis and chronic intestinal obstruction
    i. Sprue
    j. Hyperperistalsis
    k. Dysentery
    l. Steatorrhea
    m. Cystic fibrosis of pancreas
    n. Giardiasis
2. Excessive use of mineral oil
3. Cardiovascular disease
4. Advanced age
5. Prematurity, and feeding problems in infants

III. *Inadequate Utilization or Storage*
1. Diabetes mellitus
2. Advanced diseases of kidney, liver, or pancreas
3. Hypothyroidism
4. Antibiotic therapy
5. Malignancy

IV. *Increased Requirements*
1. Hyperthyroidism
2. Fever
3. Physical exertion
4. Pregnancy
5. Lactation
6. Environmental extremes
7. Rapid growth
8. Certain therapeutic regimens
9. After surgical procedures
10. Injuries
11. Certain toxic agents
12. Burns
13. Convalescence
14. Infections

V. *Increased Loss or Excretion*
1. Polyuria, such as from large quantities of fluid postoperatively
2. Blood loss
3. Negative nitrogen balance
4. Lactation

Refer to I. 12h in the preceding chart, which tells us that a baby on a formula (a substitute for breast milk, which has no substitute) needs orange juice to protect him against Vitamin C deficiency. Breast milk is an adequate source of the vitamin; it is also an adequate source of pyridoxine (Vitamin B6). That distinction was not known at the time the medical journals reprinted this chart, and for that ignorance one baby paid the price in permanent brain damage. The child, formula fed, had been born with a tendency to convulsions, which did not respond to treatment, and ultimately, brain damage occurred and, with it, permanent mental retardation. The convulsions were traced to an unfortunate coincidence of two factors: the baby was born with a high requirement for Vitamin B6; and the amount of the vitamin available in the formula was low.

It is my philosophy that insurance is not less valuable because so many people never have occasion to collect on it; and dietary insurance—which is really the reason for the use of organ meats, brewer's yeast, wheat germ, and vitamin supplements—is never a waste of effort and expense. These remarks can be applied to the generous protein intake previously recommended. Protein, in any quantity beyond the need of the body for it, as such, is converted into glycogen, the reserve sugar supply of the body. This type of fuel, as the reader now knows, is normally drawn on as needed, does not normally flood the blood with sudden increments of sugar that trigger pancreatic reaction. It is long-lasting fuel, distinct from "quick energy." Protein, which means of "first importance," is also vital to liver structure and function, and I have already pointed out that the role of the liver in hypoglycemia may be as critical as that of the pancreas.

The female reader should not quickly scan these lines and as quickly forget them, for what is not being said is as important as what is being discussed. The liver, as an example of what has been omitted, is the key organ in control of female hormone activity. Female (estrogenic) hormone has been labeled as capable of causing cancer, and this labeling was done by a federal agency that then proceeded to encourage its use in birth control pills! The well-nourished liver copes with female hormone, whether it is introduced via medication or self-manufactured. There are women who manufacture excessive amounts of female hormone, and there are nutritionists who have reason to believe that the function of the well-nourished liver is the key to control of such excessive estrogenic hormone activity, and, therefore, to control of premenstrual tension, painful menstruation, cystic mastitis, fibroid uterine tumors, and endometriosis.

The fats in the diet are today the center of research and controversy that are much too complex for discussion here. Many physicians are committed to persuading their patients to avoid or sharply reduce the intake of animal fat, avoid foods containing cholesterol, and raise the intake of vegetable fats—all this on the premise that (a) cholesterol creates deposits on the walls of the arteries, thereby initiating arteriosclerosis and associated coronary thrombosis, and that (b) reducing the amount of cholesterol in the diet will eliminate these diseases.

This thesis ignores some ugly but pertinent facts:

A. Dr. Michael DeBakey, well-known heart surgeon, has flatly stated that he found in a study of 1700 patients with atherosclerotic disease "no definite correlation between serum cholesterol levels and the nature and extent of atherosclerotic disease." Let it be emphasized that he remarks, ". . . the majority of patients in this group had serum cholesterol values within the accepted normal range for Americans."*

B. Animals that never eat animal fat or cholesterol have developed advanced hardening of the arteries—among them, the celebrated gorilla in the Chicago zoo.

C. Vegetarians who have avoided all foods high in cholesterol and all sources of animal fats have still developed arteriosclerosis and coronary thrombosis.

D. The Masais, in Africa, magnificent specimens of humanity, live on a diet extraordinarily rich in milk, blood, and meat. Coronary heart disease is practically nonexistent among them.

E. The incidence of coronary thrombosis associated with arteriosclerosis is much lower in Tucson, Arizona, than in New York City, although the Arizona diet has at least as much animal fat and cholesterol in it and probably, with the Western love for meat, more.

* H. E. Garret *et al.*, "Serum Cholesterol Values in Patients Treated Surgically for Atherosclerosis," *Journal of the American Medical Association*, Vol. 189 (August 31, 1964), pp. 655–669.

F. Two-thirds of the cholesterol in the body is manufactured in the body itself; it does not come from the diet. Perhaps this is the wisdom of the body, greater than that of the diet-tamperers, for cholesterol is essential to life, being the basis for sex hormones and for bile fluid. We can do without neither.

G. All the experiments that have been interpreted as proving that a low intake of cholesterol and animal fat reduces the incidence of heart attacks have had an uncontrolled variable: the subjects were—many of them for possibly the first time—eating balanced, planned nutrition. This is a dietary change as drastic as restriction of intake of fat and cholesterol, and there has been no way to measure its influence.

H. The studies made of the relationship between diet and the health of the arteries and heart are studies of sickness, not of health; studies of the failures, not the successes. In any old-age home, one will find eighty- and even ninety-year-old people who are contentedly eating substantial amounts of fatty meat, fatty gravies, butter, and eggs. Should we not—which we do not—ponder their health and survival, rather than concentrate on autopsies?

I. For every country that eats vegetable fats and little cholesterol and has a lower incidence of heart and artery disease than ours, there is one which eats animal fats and much cholesterol and still escapes circulatory troubles. Why ignore such countries, as so many studies do, on the apparent premise that these are merely facts which should not be allowed to interfere with a beautifully integrated theory?

J. There is clear evidence that the amount of cholesterol present is not the significant factor in arteriosclerosis. More important is the form in which it appears. One cholesterol "package" delivers its burden in the blood. The other carries the cholesterol package to the liver, where it is routed out of the body. Thus much more important than your cholesterol level is the amount of low-density lipoprotein, which is the mischief maker in the blood, versus the content of high-density lipoprotein, which carries cholesterol away.

K. In communities where the water is "soft" (low in mineral values), circulatory disorders and coronary thrombosis are more frequent than in hard-water areas.

The situation cannot be summed up because it is too confused. A conservative statement was made by the author in a national broadcast, some thirty years ago:

> Hardening of the arteries and coronary thrombosis are not a linear question of A plus B equals C, or you plus fat and cholesterol equal hardening of the arteries and coronary heart disease. If this were true, the diet could be used to predict susceptibility, and it can't. After all, women may share their husbands' meals, but don't share the susceptibility to heart attacks, which is dominated by the males. The tendency is the product of a multiordinate equation in which the diet is only one of a number of variables, and many other factors, from environmental stresses to the genes, play a determining role. Overeating may well prove to be the dominant role of diet in these diseases, and if any dietary factor has even a claim to an important relationship to circulatory disorders and heart disease, it may well turn out to be the dietary carbohydrates— especially, the abuse of sugar.

Nothing has happened in the years since that broadcast to mandate a change in the statement. On that basis, the reader will not anticipate that this text will urge abstention from eggs, drowning oneself in vegetable fats, or switching entirely from whole milk to nonfat. Too radical a change such as this in the diet, on the basis of present evidence, is a journey into the uncharted—with unpredictable results.

There *are* recommendations that can safely be made if one wishes to use fats in a sane way that may contribute to well-being. Limited use of vegetable fats is reasonable; excessive use can be dangerous. In the previous edition of this book the use of margarine was recommended because the American diet has been significantly deficient in factors supplied by vegetable fats. At that time, there was no information available on the dangers of margarine. Subsequently, some disconcerting actions of "partially hydrogenated fats," such as are used in margarine, were established. Hindsight is 20/20, but I think that you deserve this explanation of a significant change in my recommendations. I now employ linseed oil, safflower oil, and sesame oil as sources of polyunsaturated fat, and no longer recommend margarine. Some of the vegetable oils on the market also have undesirable additives, such as BHT and BHA. If the oil contained enough Vitamin E, artificial preservatives would not be needed, but I have learned that one practice of the vegetable oil industry is extraction of the Vitamin E for sale to vitamin-concentrate manufacturers, thereby compelling the use of the synthetic antioxidants as preservatives. I strongly suggest that you buy vegetable oils in health-food stores, rather than in the supermarket, and that you do not overdose. Since we do not know how much Vitamin E remains in the oil, as the intake of this type of fat is raised, the amount of Vitamin E supplement should go up proportionately, for an oversupply of unsaturated fat can create a Vitamin E deficiency. One baby being fed fat intravenously died because his physician was unaware of this relationship, and while no extreme penalty would result for an adult taking slight overdoses of such an oil, since there are Vitamin E supplies in other foods, there appears to be no point in taking unnecessary chances in a nutritional world where so many hazards are inescapable. It should be remembered that the overprocessing of carbohydrates, previously discussed, removes more than 90 percent of the Vitamin E from grains; and most of the vitamin that escapes this raping of the grain is destroyed by added measures like the bleaching of flour.

Polyunsaturated fats, it should be explained, have the ability to unite chemically with hydrogen (hence "unsaturated" with hydrogen). If hydrogen cannot be chemically inserted in the fat molecule, it is then considered "saturated." Most animal fats are highly saturated; most vegetable fats are not. The significance of this distinction lies in two actions of vegetable fat: they do not lend themselves to formation of fat deposits that resist reducing; and they do not ordinarily raise blood cholesterol but tend to reduce it. The last statement is not inconsistent with what has been said before. Elevated blood cholesterol is no more desirable than abnormally elevated blood sugar.

The reference to fat deposits does not do justice to the phenomenon observed in overweight subjects who adopt the low-sugar, low-carbohydrate diet as a reducing plan. If the fat in such a diet is unsaturated, astonishing amounts of protein and fat can be taken while weight loss continues unabated.* If some of the fat is saturated, the low-

* Recent research in stubborn cases of obesity indicates that the type of unsaturated fat employed to aid reducing with a low-carbohydrate diet is important. The vegetable oils that the public considers to be polyunsaturated are actually not. These are omega 6 oils. Omega 3 oils are, for sound biochemical reasons,

carbohydrate reducing diet is much less effective, even though the calorie intake is the same. Such a reducing diet—low carbohydrate, high protein, and high fat (with 20 percent of the fat calories from the unsaturated form)—also has striking effectiveness in causing weight loss in problem areas ordinarily not responsive to the conventional reducing diet. The loss in inches seems all out of proportion to the loss in weight, an added dividend much appreciated by those who bulge in the wrong places; but this kind of redistribution of body fat also takes place with such a diet, even when weight reduction is not needed and not achieved.

In terms of general health, not hypoglycemia, a reasonable use of edible-grade linseed oil may be beneficial. So may the use of cod liver oil, which is now available deodorized or deodorized with peppermint added. These oils convey benefits not obtainable from ordinary vegetable oil. Similarly, there are dividends from the use of oily fish—trout, mackerel, anchovies, sardines, and salmon—as a source of protein in the diet. Among them, from the type of oil contained in such fish, is very real protection against hardening of the arteries and heart attacks. Such fish can be substituted for any other protein recommended in the hypoglycemia diets you will find in this text.

This brief survey of protein, fat, and carbohydrate in the diet should not be taken as an education in nutrition. It is intended as a blueprint of the pathway toward sensible nutrition. If it has stimulated your desire to learn more, the library is filled with texts on the subject, which are valuable when you learn to separate scientific information from propaganda masquerading as such. Nutrition texts that eulogize enriched

more effective. The most inexpensive and widely available variety of omega 3 oils is linseed oil. One must be careful to avoid the commercial grade of linseed oil, which is used in paints. The edible grade is sold at some health-food stores. A daily intake of one to two tablespoonfuls of edible-grade linseed oil has markedly improved the success of reducers on a low-carbohydrate diet. This biochemical magic is slow in developing, though, and may require from six weeks to two months. When using this type of fatty acid, it is also necessary to use antioxidants. Without antioxidants, the linseed oil in the body may be subject to deterioration, the same type it would suffer if stored in the pantry in a warm place. The most effective and easily available antioxidants can be found combined in one capsule in a number of brands. Regular use of such a supplement yields other dividends as well, including an anti-aging effect.

white bread as nutritionally equivalent to whole wheat reflect, if not direct commercial influence, at least indoctrination rather than education. Books that insist that all Americans are well nourished, need no special criteria in selecting a balanced diet, and need no vitamin supplements present bias and prejudice in the guise of information. Texts that belabor food faddism must be carefully scanned. In his day, Freud was labeled as a quack by his colleagues; Hans Berger, who brought us the electroencephalogram, was rejected as a faddist and informed that medicine would never toy with such electronic cultism; and the physician who proposed the concept of psychosomatic medicine was accused of dabbling in quackery and was laughed off the platform at one of the medical societies. The AMA itself declared in 1917 that doctors were too smart to fall into the trap of believing that deficiencies in vitamins caused a number of diseases. Even statements on nutrition from major universities must be examined in the context of the grants on which these nutrition departments function; some professors are curiously unwilling to admit that any criticism of highly processed foods may have a basis in fact.

If these remarks are startling, please remember that you have been reading a book on the lag in medicine, which has permitted millions of people to suffer unnecessary torture from an unrecognized, untreated, unfashionable disorder: hypoglycemia.

# 5. From Emotional Disturbances to Low Blood Sugar to Increased Emotional Disorder

That low blood sugar can change personality and behavior is easy to accept when one remembers how dependent brain and nervous system are on a constant, stable (if small) supply of sugar. Three times each minute, the brain completes a fantastic series of chemical reactions (the Krebs cycle) in which sugar is converted into energy.

Less easy to comprehend is the pathway by which emotional disturbances can cause low blood sugar and so begin a vicious circle. That is really the story of man's two brains, which is fascinating and yet largely unappreciated by most laymen. Man's outer brain, like the shell of a walnut, encloses an inner brain, like the walnut itself. The outer brain (cortex, which means "bark") is the thinking brain. It developed relatively late in man's evolution. The inner brain, the thalamus, is man's ancient nerve center. It is the primitive brain with which the baby, in whom the cortex is largely undeveloped, is born. It is the selfish, grasping brain. It is the home of "I love that. Gimmee it. Get out of my way. I don't care. I hate you. I'll kill you if you block me." The outer brain, developing gradually, exercises control over the rebel. An animal turns into a human being as this control is exerted. "I want that. Get out of my way!" becomes "Yes, I'd like another piece, but are you sure you're really not hungry?"

Seated in the thalamic (emotional) brain is control over many of the autonomic functions of the body. This relieves us of the responsibility to remember to breathe, to keep the heart beating, to change the circulation when there is a change in external temperature, or, for that matter, to dilate the pupils when the light grows dim.

For her own good reasons, Nature has seen to it that virtually all stimulation that reaches the thinking brain must first pass through the emotional brain. Have you ever said, "The more I thought about it, the more angry I became!"? That sentence recognizes the duality of man's brain. It also recognizes that there is a point at which the thinking brain cannot control the emotional brain. Finally, it reflects an error, because the thinking did not fan the anger. It merely justified releasing it. All stimuli reaching the thinking brain must first travel through the emotional center. The thought was tinged with red anger when it began. In fact, there is no such thing as unemotional, objective thought; the anatomy of the mind makes this impossible.

A quarrel between these two brains can cause low blood sugar, which will then disturb both brains. Let's see how. Let us assume that you have your brother-in-law living with you. This is bad enough in a three-room apartment, but he is also an intolerable boor. He swills his soup, gargles his coffee, had bad breath, tells foul jokes, never shaves, and rarely bathes. Your thalamic brain says, "Throw the bum out!" Your cortex replies, "He *is* my husband's brother!" The thalamic brain, cunning, replies, "No marriage vow 'for better or worse' ever included my husband's family." The cortex answers, "Logic won't take care of this. He's my husband's brother." The thalamic brain doesn't stop trying. It becomes irritated when the boor breathes, though he obviously must. It makes you edgy. You find your fingers slipping as you pour his hot coffee, as though the thalamus were determined to broil him alive—which it is. Ultimately, the time comes when the cortex, in self-preservation, must rebel against the constant bickering with the emotional brain. "I can't go on with these complaints," it says, "when there is really nothing I can do about the situation. So I'm not going to recognize you! As far as I'm concerned, and where my brother-in-law is concerned, my thalamic brain doesn't exist." At this point, the psychiatrist would say you had pushed the resentment down into your subconscious and persuaded yourself on the thinking level that there are redeeming features about a man with halitosis, dirty feet, and vile table manners.

In the thalamic brain, there is a will to do something, denied by the cortex, which has exclusive control over the voluntary muscles. However dearly the emotional brain would like to nudge you into throwing something at your constant guest, it cannot make you lift a finger without the cooperation of the thinking brain. So that will-to-do is now burning briskly in the thalamus—with nowhere to go and nothing *voluntary* to be done. Since it cannot escape "upward," through the thinking brain, it turns downward, for there lies the domain of the emotional brain. That ball of fire must find its outlet. What will it be?

The thalamus may choose to overstimulate nerves and muscles so that you have a tremor that makes it difficult for you to pass a dish to your brother-in-law or so you suffer with painful cramps when he has been near you. It may decide to give you rapid beating of the heart with extra systoles (a sensation of skipping and added beats) that will drive you into going fearfully to a cardiac specialist in search of a nonexistent heart disease. It may choose to stimulate the mechanism that controls the production of stomach acid, so that you develop an ulcer. Or, if that is your particular weakness, it may decide to overstimulate the entire adreno-sympathetic system, from which all sorts of phenomena will develop. The response of the adrenal gland will keep the entire body poised for fight or flight, when in fact you can do neither, and this may send your blood pressure soaring. Adrenal hormones will give you attacks of anxiety, which to you will seem unprovoked. The hormones will draw sugar (glycogen) from your reserves in the liver and feed it to the blood, and this in turn will induce the pancreas to manufacture insulin to keep the sugar level down to normal. (Here is the start of the process that leads to low blood sugar.) By this time, what with anxiety, increased blood pressure, a racing and skipping heart, indigestion, and the penalties of low blood sugar, the emotional brain will have reached the cortex with an unmistakable message which that brain will not be able to ignore, a message reading: "If you do not agree to do something about this situation, I'm going to keep both of us from functioning."

You now can clearly see the pattern: it begins with anxiety and tension, which lead to low blood sugar. But low blood sugar of itself will ring an alarm in the body, and the adrenal gland will respond in an effort to raise the sugar level. In this effort, hormones are produced that create anxiety—and around you go. Unfortunately, long after the brother-in-law has gone, the pressure has subsided, and the heart has quieted, the low blood sugar may remain. You will by then have nibbled on enough sweets to make the pancreas hypersensitive, ruin your figure, lose your spouse, and contribute to the support of a few psychiatrists.

# 6.   Hypoglycemia and the Spirits

Modern psychology, which has so dexterously solved the problems of crime, war, and marital infidelity, has not hesitated in isolating the root causes of alcoholism, which turn out to be one: a need to escape the harshness of reality. It has been suggested by cynics that this is an analysis that raises more questions than it answers. Why this particular escape from reality, why this rocky, forbidding, lonely, vicious circle? Why not movies, blondes, or even marijuana?

There are those who ridicule the definition of alcoholism as a disorder of emotional origin. If it were, they point out, some pattern of personality unique to the alcoholic, some aberration of the psyche that makes the first drink one too many should be identifiable. Yet there is no personality profile of the drunkard that could not be fitted to many nondrinkers. These dissenters say it's a physical disease, but that explanation is faulty, too, for if alcoholism is a physical disorder, there should be some metabolic characteristic of an alcoholic that is peculiar to his breed. One such biochemical aberration *has* been identified.

Still a third theory is held by some very practical scientists who insist that compulsive drinking is no more a disease than lying or thieving. To them, an alcoholic is simply somebody who drinks too much, gives lip service to his desire to dry out, and won't stop.

These are not academic arguments about a problem of a small minority. There are at least five million victims of alcoholism in the United States, which means that more than twenty-five million people, ranging from employers to relatives and from friends to co-workers, are directly or indirectly involved in the problem. This means that anything even remotely helpful to alcoholics is worthy of investigation. And yet there are two promising leads that have been neglected, perhaps because psychiatry has dominated this field and both clues lie in the area of the purely physical.

Although this subject is obviously one that may drive warring scientists to drink, all the agencies that deal with it do agree on the drinker's need of nutritional support. From Alcoholics Anonymous to the Salvation Army, regular meals are always part of a prescription that includes faith in a deity, social support, and the finding of a purpose and a reward in sobriety.

Unfortunately, there has been a tacit assumption behind all efforts to persuade alcoholics to eat regularly that what is considered good nutrition for the nondrinker is automatically good diet for the drunkard, unless he has so far descended the ladder of deficiency that he is a victim of one of the diseases of malnourishment—beriberi, pellagra, or cirrhosis of the liver.* In those cases, he is plied with vitamins by mouth and by injection, coupled with an intensive course of high-protein diet therapy.

Yet the proposition that alcoholics have the same dietary needs as nondrinkers rests on no evidence at all. As a matter of fact, the only significant evidence available points to a completely opposite possibility: that within the alcoholic population there is a group, perhaps a substantial minority, which is involved in either or both of two nutritional problems, and that solution of these dietetic problems may allow a compulsive drinker to escape from his trap.

The research that raises one of these possibilities was performed by Professor Roger Williams, of the Clayton Biochemical Foundation, who is the former president of the American Chemical Society. It began with animals being given free access to alcohol, a step that promptly exhibited the whole spectrum of behavior one would encounter in a human population afforded the same opportunity. Some of the animals abstained. Some were occasional drinkers. A percentage were true dipsomaniacs, going on periodic binges, with intervening periods of sobriety. A group became confirmed animal alcoholics, taking as much as 40 percent of their calories from alcohol.

Dr. Williams, long preoccupied with man's biochemical differences, made a study of the chemistry of the bodies of the obsessive animal drinkers and found that those who were not able to stop drinking *did differ chemically* from the teetotalers. They showed abnormally high requirements for certain dietary essentials, particularly vitamins—re-

* Cirrhosis may not always be a deficiency disease. It may be a result of the toxic effect of alcohol.

quirements so high that the ordinary "well-balanced" animal diet fell short of meeting their needs. The resulting deficiency was expressed in a perverted form by addiction to alcohol. As the intake of these nutrients was raised to satisfy their requirements, the appetite of the animals for alcohol began to fall and sometimes vanished entirely. Williams was able to conclude that these responses showed inborn metabolic differences, present in the animals at birth and creating abnormally great nutritional requirements.

If he had stopped his work at that point, it would still have been a basis for testing a new approach to human alcoholism, but this scientist knows well that you cannot write of mice and men without testing men. This he did, though the number of subjects involved was too few for definitive conclusions. He reported that the human drinkers tested responded as the animals had, and after high dosages of vitamins, were able to refuse to drink, or even to take the first drink and yet refuse the second.

If you are naive enough to hope that other workers picked up the trail, investigated the nutritional needs of alcoholics, and tried the treatment on subjects found suitable, you are not aware of the propaganda campaign that has labeled vitamin supplements as placebos (mere inert vehicles for the power of suggestion) and that suggests that all Americans, at all economic levels, are beautifully nourished and need no supplements of any kind. The fact is that human beings are remarkably unalike biochemically, and these differences extend to their eating habits, which range from the abominable to the superb, and to their dietary needs. At any rate, Williams' work, reported in his *Nutrition and Alcoholism* (University of Oklahoma Press, 1951), is gathering dust in the library. Why?

Oddly enough, there is a parallel between his findings and certain observations concerning mice genetically subject to "audiogenic seizures." These are convulsions induced by exposure to a high-pitched sound. The trait is inborn, but it can be modified by changes in the animals' diets, something that was learned by giving the mice free access to a group of vitamins. They selected thiamin (B1) as the one vitamin of which they apparently simply couldn't eat enough. They raised their intake by a factor of seven or eight, far beyond their "requirement" as set in the lab manuals. The audiogenic seizures diminished in intensity, duration, and frequency until they faded out entirely. The same approach was made to stammering in human beings, the theory being that this disorder, another of the many long considered to be of purely emotional origin, might in some cases also be the product of a nervous system overreactive because of an unsatisfied (and extraordinarily high) requirement for Vitamin B1. Benefits have come to some stammerers treated in this way, and the parallel with alcoholism is inescapable, for in the treatment of such speech impediments, proponents of the emotional theory have dominated the field, and those who have speculated on possible physical causes have been viewed with some suspicion.

At about the time that Williams' book was published Dr. Wolfgang Seligmann and I were deep in research with the problem of low blood sugar. Although the main thrust of the investigation was aimed at the relationship between hypoglycemia and allergy (particularly asthma), several alcoholics were encountered who, in response to the high-vitamin dosage and the frequent, small, high-protein, high-fat meals, which together constitute the nutritional treatment for low blood sugar, had responded with an ability to reject alcohol entirely or to stop after taking the first drink. The improvement was attributed to a normalization of faulty carbohydrate (starch-sugar) metabolism, but Williams' theory raised an equally interesting question: was the response a by-product of helping the alcoholics meet extraordinarily high nutritional requirements? After all, whether hypoglycemia or unsatisfied nutritional requirements can cause alcoholism, either explanation frees the drinker from the charge that he is unwilling to stop, for alcoholism inevitably will worsen low blood sugar and intensify nutritional deficiencies—vicious circles from which no one, unaided, could possibly escape.

Before I discuss the undoubted relationship of low blood sugar to alcoholism, let me pause to scold those who have ignored or arbitrarily rejected Williams' thesis. Those who have attempted to identify a unique pattern of personality or metabolism in the human alcoholic should at least be scientifically tolerant of an effort to identify in these sufferers a group whose abnormal dietary requirements mark them apart from other drinkers and from the general population.

The role of hypoglycemia in this problem has received equally little attention. Hypoglycemia *induced* by drinking has been reported, particularly in patients with a poor dietary history, but why has no one studied the opposite and provocative possibility—that low blood sugar itself can cause compulsive drinking? Yet there is evidence that it can and does—and not infrequently—evidence that, like Williams' theory, has been ignored in the apparent hope that it will somehow go away. Possibly this is so because we are always looking for *the* cure; it is so much simpler than looking for many. We prattle about *the* cure for cancer, which is not a single disease. *The* cure for alcoholism is a tempting simplification. Actually, controlling hypoglycemia has been followed in some hundreds of cases of compulsive drinking by voluntary and sustained abstention.

More than eight in every ten hypoglycemics have a ravenous appetite for sweets, which illustrates an aberration of the "wisdom of the body," since the overactive pancreas, which spurs the desire for sweets, will be restimulated when sugar is eaten. Such a strong desire for sugar is also characteristic of a group of alcoholics—but not confined to them—who alternate between periods of sobriety and abysmal intoxication. The quantities of candy they can consume while sober are almost unbelievable and offer a clue to low blood sugar, which, extraordinarily enough, has been overlooked. *Life* magazine once told the story of Pappy Boyington, the famous ace of World War II, who fought his own battle with drinking. His wife was quoted as saying that he could, over a sober weekend, eat pounds of candy. Periodic drinkers have been known to eat five pounds of chocolates in twenty-four hours—always when sober, never when drinking. Such compulsive craving literally pleads for sugar-tolerance tests, but if such tests are made and hypoglycemia *is* found, it is inevitably regarded as the result rather than the possible cause of alcoholism.

Then, too, as has been explained elsewhere, the test may be misinterpreted because of a basic error in our "normal range" for blood sugar. Blood sugars within this "normal range" have reportedly produced clear symptoms of hypoglycemia, and alcoholics in this group demonstrated a mounting resistance to compulsive drinking as diet and vitamin treatment was used to bring the low blood sugar under control. Gyland remarks that he successfully treated 600 hypoglycemic patients of whom a majority would have evaded proper diagnosis and treatment, which, indeed, would have happened if blood sugar levels within the "normal range" had been accepted as the criteria of normalcy. Among these were 20 alcoholics, and most of these drinkers were able to break their habit once hypoglycemia had been properly treated!

Gyland's paper, printed in a Brazilian medical journal, in Portuguese, certainly stirred no wave of interest in the relationship between hypoglycemia and alcoholism. The paper should have—but didn't—induced psychiatrists and psychologists to take a second look at some of their "neurotic" patients; it should have moved allergists to check blood sugars in asthmatics, but it didn't. It joined Williams' book in dusty and "innocuous desuetude."

As cancer in mice exposed to cigarette smoke proves only that mice should not smoke, so successful treatment of alcoholism by successful treatment of hypoglycemia does not prove that low blood sugar *causes* alcoholism. All we can say is that there is a *possible* causal relationship. How strong that possibility is, we shall never learn if these observations continue to mold in the library. Speaking of mold, it would seem that we are at the same stage as Alexander Fleming when he realized that mold seemed to have the power to retard the growth of bacteria. His colleagues fought him and his theory with bitter skepticism. The result was that some fifteen years were to pass before Fleming's chance observation was recognized as the discovery of penicillin and then could be applied to help suffering humanity. Over thirty-five years have passed since Gyland published his study. The Seligmann and Fredericks research was reported back in 1952. How long will it be before someone again follows this path to determine if there is a reward for alcoholics at its end? It *is* there. We need only determine to how many alcoholics this treatment may logically be applied. It must be remembered that *all* alcoholics are subject to low blood sugar, if not as cause, then as a result of the substitution of alcohol for food, and that treating hypoglycemia may benefit tremendously any compulsive drinker, even if cure of the compulsion does not follow—which it may!

It has been said that honest men profit when thieves fall out. When scientists disagree, a chasm opens into which the helpless layman may fall, and the only sensible path for him to choose is the one that appears safest, if not the most promising. In the case of treating hypoglycemia in an effort to help alcoholics, there is no question of safety: no one has ever been hurt by a good diet coupled with Vitamin B Complex supplements. That, though, does not make the way any easier for the patient who is determined to find out (a) if he has low blood sugar and (b) whether, if present, it is the cause of his particular variety of alcoholism. If he does succeed in arriving at a glucose-tolerance test, he may still be in trouble, for he must then convince many practitioners that his hypoglycemia is not necessarily a *result* of his drinking but a potential cause.

These difficulties have already been discussed, but a question remains: why is the test so often misinterpreted, so that a diagnosis of normal blood sugar is rendered when hypoglycemia is actually present? The next chapter tells the fascinating, if dismaying, story of norms that are actually abnormal because they are derived from sick people considered normal because their state of health is average.

# 7. Abnormal Norms

Averages are deceiving, and statisticians early learn to distrust them. After all, a man's *average* temperature is comfortable when he has one foot in a bucket of dry ice and the other in an oxygen-hydrogen flame! Averages are deceiving, too, if your sample population is too small. What conclusions are properly drawn if the first hundred people you meet in New York City are Italians or Democrats or carry switchblade knives? Averages mislead if your sample is unbalanced. The "average income" in a group of one hundred Americans that happens to include four billionaires would not be reflected in the tax returns of one hundred of them!

Of all the traps within the concept of "average" none is more misleading than the temptation to confuse *average* with *normal*. In a universe of sick people, the averages will be considered as norms; the true abnormality would be good health. That is our situation, and what is worse is our blindness to it.

The outsider is quick to perceive the difficulty. A Norwegian physician once remarked to an American colleague: "Your physicians label women as 'well nourished' who in Norway would be put under treatment for nutritional anemia!" Sometimes, time itself offers a perspective. In 1932 a pediatrician examined the blood chemistry of thousands of newborn children to set standards for norms in infants. For years these were used as a yardstick by which to judge the health of a newborn baby, but if an infant of today did not surpass these standards, he would be placed under treatment for malnourishment!

Now consider the norms applied to you, as an adult, for red blood cells, for hemoglobin, for white cells, for body temperature . . . for any of the body phenomena the physicians appraise. From what kinds of people were the samples derived for these norms? Sick people obviously were excluded. One cannot set up standards for the healthy based on the chemistries of patients with heart disease, cancer, collagen disorders, auto-immune diseases, hardening of the arteries, arthritis, and other gross sicknesses. But were people with allergies excluded? With too many colds? Fatigability, decayed teeth, postnasal drip, virus infections, frequent sore throats, indigestion, constipation? Obviously not. Such people are average; thereby normal; thereby healthy!

It occurred to a competent medical researcher that it might be useful to reexamine the standards by establishing the norms for a group of *truly healthy* people. His first task, obviously, was to find them—not an easy accomplishment in a country where the ability to walk upright if the wind is blowing in the right direction is counted as evidence of superb well-being. The investigator found his subjects in a group of dental students. Most professional schools insist that applicants be in good health on the pragmatic grounds that it is wasteful to pour expensive, subsidized education into someone who will not be well enough to practice. From the original group, the physician gained his first set of "norms," which unsurprisingly fell within the ranges listed in the medical textbooks as characteristic of "healthy American adults."

Having established these ranges, the researcher now began to drop from the group those who did not measure up to a stricter definition of good health. Thus he excluded those with loose teeth, with too many colds, with a touch of sinus trouble, with a bit of allergy, with a little constipation. And as the group shrank in numbers and became an elite selection of genuinely healthy, "symptomless, signless" men, the ranges established in the various categories—red cells, hemoglobin, blood sugar, etc.—began to change. The more select the group and the more it truly approached genuine good health, the more the ranges shrank. For example, let us say that the original population showed a fasting blood sugar ranging from 60 to 120 milligrams percent, which is what the textbooks label as "normal." As the group shrank in numbers and gained in well-being, those figures narrowed to a range of, let us say, 68 to 87.

From such a trend, one may make a good, educated guess at its direction, provided the original group were large enough. It is obvious that the blood sugars would ultimately wind up as a fixed figure, varying only very slightly from individual to individual. Statisticians calculated this as 76 to 77 milligrams percent of sugar in the blood (fasting), plus or minus a small percentage of error in the determinations.

If this ostensibly minor declaration were finally accepted as the truly normal fasting blood sugar in truly normal people, the medical destiny of millions would be changed. Those who are now being told they are healthy will accurately be relabeled as pre-diabetic. Those who have been assured they do not have hypoglycemia to explain their "emotional" symptoms, alcoholism, or drug addiction will be reappraised as victims of low blood sugar! That reappraisal, though, cannot rest on one single determination of the blood sugar level when the stomach is empty. It cannot even be determined by a test of blood sugar at the very moment when the patient is having an attack that seems to result from low blood sugar. These remarks, which seem more fit for the medical forum than for a book for the layman, are needed. Not only is the medical profession inclined to look for anything but low blood sugar, not only are the "normal range" figures misleading, but the method of testing, the time of testing, and the interpretation are likely to lead to wrong conclusions.

Let me explain:

1. A person with blood sugar levels within normal range (as now interpreted) may still have low blood sugar . . . low for *him*, and contributing to his "neurosis," compulsive drinking, drug addiction, or inability to get along with his wife.

2. Blood sugar levels may be within "normal range," however defined, even during an attack, and yet be responsible for the attack.

3. No reliable negative conclusions can safely be drawn from one or two determinations of blood sugar levels, whether taken when the person has been fasting or after he has eaten. My interest in blood sugar is in its dynamics. I think like a banker, who is not so much interested in the amount of money in your account at the moment as he is in the record of how you handle it.

4. Little recognized—even by some of those who are concerned with sugar levels in the blood, such as diabetic specialists—is the fact that when the blood sugar drops as little as 2 milligrams percent below the normal for the person, a profound glandular compensation may start, in an effort by the body to restore the sugar level to normal before the brain and nervous system are affected adversely. This, the beginning of the process that, by stimulating the adrenal gland, leads to the distressing anxiety which hypoglycemics suffer, may ultimately lead to diabe-

tes. It is for this reason that Seale Harris, MD, a pioneer in the treatment of diabetes and in the recognition of low blood sugar as a disease entity, wrote that "the hypoglycemic of today is the diabetic of tomorrow." This, of course, makes it even more imperative that hypoglycemia be promptly recognized and competently treated. No one, and certainly no practitioner of medicine, is entitled to brush off a blood sugar reading as being "only a couple of points below normal," yet the comment is appallingly common.

5. No blood sugar level, whenever it falls, can safely be labeled as "low normal" when it is associated with symptoms that could be caused by low blood sugar. The medical axiom must be: "If in doubt, treat." Let the response to treatment make the diagnosis; never let the laboratory insist that the sick patient is well.

6. Tests of blood sugar over a period of two to three hours are not adequate. Some people do not show the signs of hypoglycemia until six hours after they have been challenged with a dose of sugar. A six-hour test is ordered by the competent physician.

7. If the physician wishes to try to avoid the prolonged series of blood sugar tests, there is one shortcut that may be used, but it must be employed and interpreted with caution. It is a simple technique that takes less than an hour and that may prove a useful screening device.

Basically, the test calls for a determination of the fasting blood sugar level before breakfast. The patient is then instructed to eat his normal breakfast, and the test is repeated forty-five minutes to one hour later. If the blood sugar at that time has not risen 50 milligrams percent or more above the fasting level, the patient is hypoglycemic, and this is true even though the initial and the second readings fall within "normal range."

This may be compared with the long test in which many blood sugar levels are determined over a six-hour period, after sugar has been fed as a challenge to the pancreas. Here the physician is screening the results for three phenomena:

A. A failure of the sugar levels to rise as high as they should which would argue for faulty absorption or, which is more likely, overproduction of insulin.

B. The converse: excessive elevation of sugar levels, which may indicate a pre-diabetic or a diabetic state.

C. Elevation of the sugar levels at the end of the test, or the converse: a drop below the original fasting level. If the drop is 20 milligrams percent or more below the fasting level, hypoglycemia is confirmed. If the drop is 10 to 20 milligrams percent, a state of pre-hypoglycemia is suggested. If there is an elevation of the sugar levels, diabetes again is diagnosed.

It is the length, expense, and discomfort of the long test that have contributed to its unpopularity and certainly tended to suppress the physician's index of suspicion for hypoglycemia. Diabetes, after all, is much easier to identify, for even a single blood or urine sample may give a leading clue, though even then, the long test becomes mandatory. The physician is aware of the predictability of diabetes when there is a family history of it. The treatment for it has a certain drama. The protracted therapy with diet and vitamins, required for hypoglycemia, has very little of the glamour of medicine on the march.

The question raised by the short test and interpretation is simple: is it accurate? Is there reliability in its predictions that the long test will or will not, as the case may be, reveal the presence of low blood sugar? One can at least say for it that it doesn't seem to give false positives. If this brief test, with its two blood samplings, labels you as a hypoglycemic, the longer tests are most likely to do the same. If the short test exonerates you, and yet the symptoms insistently suggest hypoglycemia, the wise physician can always order the longer procedure.

One must be sure, though, that interpretation of the long test is competent. Some physicians—and this has been observed—obtaining a final reading lower than the fasting level by 20 milligrams percent of sugar, may regard this as an insignificant drop, or choose to disregard the decline because the final figure is still within "normal range." Gyland, who treated more hypoglycemics than any other physician who has published a clinical report, is quite definite when he labels a drop below the fasting level of as little as 10 milligrams percent as meaningful. I. M. Somogyi, a peerless authority on insulin therapy, is quite definite when he remarks that a 3 milligrams percent drop in sugar levels below normal has a profound impact upon the body's stress-resisting mechanism.

To illustrate how a patient who has been given the six-hour test for low blood sugar may still be the victim of misinterpretation of abnormal norms, consider the case of a thirty-nine-year-old woman who was hospitalized because of a bleeding duodenal ulcer. She had distinct symptoms of low blood sugar: internal feelings of tremor, shaking of the extremities, episodes of pallor and clammy sweating, fatigue, anxiety, insomnia, nightmares, and difficulty in concentrating. On that basis, the physician ordered a glucose-tolerance test. She began with a fasting sugar of 60. The physician labeled it normal. She ended with a sugar level of 53 milligrams percent. "A little low," said the physician, "but not hypoglycemia." His standard for low blood sugar was any level below 50. He forgot one lesson all physicians must learn: when the laboratory insists that the patient is well, and the patient insists that she is sick, the doctor must rely on his knowledge, experience, and intuition. He forgot one lesson any real student of hypoglycemia must remember: no blood sugar is a "little low" if the patient has symptoms of low blood sugar. A consultant insisted that the patient be treated with the hypoglycemia diet, and all arguments ended; her symptoms disappeared.

The way to end the welter of argument, the debate about norms, the quarrel about techniques of testing is to make a therapeutic diagnosis, to question the presence of low blood sugar by treating it, rather than testing for it. If the symptoms disappear, the diagnosis is confirmed in the best possible way, for, as was remarked in the discussion of alcoholism, no one has ever been hurt by the good nutrition of the hypoglycemia diet and vitamin supplements. And there is precedent for therapeutic diagnosis: it has often been used in gout, where diagnosis is not firm, for there is a drug that does not affect other types of arthritis at all, but is a blessing to the gout sufferer. The medical man will feel that the exquisite pain of the condition warrants the therapeutic trial, and if the gout is relieved by the medication, he can, from the comfortable vantage point of hindsight, say: "It must have been gout. Otherwise, this medicine would not have helped." Is this procedure somehow unjustified in hypoglycemia, the total impact of which is far more devastating than pain in a big toe?

# 8. If Every Man Would Mend a Man, Then Would All Men Be Mended

He was an attorney who—for no good reason apparent to him—suffered from chronic, low-grade depression, alternating with periods of unprovoked anxiety. His family doctor, who knew him well, said it was all understandable, what with his problems with his law partner, complications in his life with his three daughters and his wife, and the chronic fatigue and zestlessness he had endured for more than five years. It all *had* to be largely emotional, for his physical examination was "essentially negative." In fact, the physician thought, he was in pretty good shape for a man of his age, working under pressures, with infrequent vacations and no opportunity for exercise.

The lawyer had persistent morning headaches, not severe enough to immobilize him but certainly capable of keeping him from functioning in the early hours. The medical man's insistence that personal problems that are headaches can be translated into physical headaches ultimately persuaded him to visit a psychiatrist, who was blunt enough to tell him that his symptoms suggested only that he was a fool to think his problems were significant. The attitude of both practitioners was: "Please take the tranquilizer when you need it, the psychoenergizer when you need a lift, and the sleeping pills when the insomnia is troublesome, and let us take care of our really sick patients."

The prescription for the sleeping pills particularly troubled the patient, for his insomnia was unpredictable. His trouble did not lie in dropping off to sleep, but in awakening in the small hours of the morning, unable to drop off again. How does one take sleeping drugs for that? The headaches continuing to torture him, he went to a diagnostician who had a reputation for his success in tracking down the sources of this common ailment. He was startled when, after some searching questions about his smoking (heavy), sweet tooth (intense), and the effects of liquor upon him (gratifying at first, terrible later), the internist insisted that he undergo a six-hour glucose-tolerance test. The graph on the next page shows his response to a dose of sugar on an empty stomach.

The curve is the type Gyland calls "pre-hypoglycemic," but the reader will remember that Gyland found that many symptoms could originate with mild low blood sugar or with the "pre-hypoglycemic state." The curve also falls into the classification of outright low blood sugar according to the criterion devised by Dr. Herman Goodman, the one-hour level not being 50 milligrams percent above the fasting level. By whatever standard his test result is judged, it clearly points to the ultimate cause of the attorney's troubles, for when he was placed on the hypoglycemia diet and was persuaded to reduce his drinking and smoking and abuse of aspirin (good for headaches but bad for sensitive patients with low blood sugar), his depression, anxiety, and headaches disappeared.

The important lesson to be learned from this history is the possible significance of *any* deviation in *any* degree from the range of blood sugar *normal for the person*. Since we rarely know what that is, we must conclude, once again, that the ultimate test of hypoglycemia is not made in the laboratory, is not determined by a textbook "normal range," and is not decided in the physician's mind. It is made at the dining table, and this is a test to which every patient with symptoms suggestive of hypoglycemia is entitled.

The next patient history concerns a young married woman with a history of diabetes on both sides of her family. For this reason, her physician had kept a careful eye on her blood sugar levels, which, from her teens on, had shown a slight tendency toward her hereditary disease. She married because she was pregnant, a situation that created bitter discord between her parents and her, and the marriage proved to be unhappy from the moment she left the altar. She lost her baby, which was stillborn and very much overweight, a tendency shown in the children of many women who subsequently develop diabetes.

What with her tensions with her parents, the stresses of her marriage, and the death of her baby, it appeared to her physician that her subsequent bouts with peptic ulcer and asthma were obviously a psychosomatic expression of her troubles, and he referred her to a psychiatric clinic operated by a religious community organization. She underwent psychotherapy for four years, during which period her marriage dissolved and both of her parents died. The worsening of her ulcer attacks and asthma seemed logically to be related to these added emotional tensions. At this point, after a two-hour glucose-tolerance test, severe diabetes was diagnosed. This reaffirmed for her psychiatrist the possible role of emotional tension in that disease, and caused her physician to place her on a strict diet, on which she cheated persistently. What with her dietary laxity and the blood-sugar-raising effect of the asthma medications she was using, control of her soaring blood sugar levels became very difficult, and the internist ultimately prescribed insulin for her. Whatever benefit this treatment yielded for her diabetes, it did nothing for her asthma and her stomach ulcer attacks, which began to increase in frequency, severity, and duration.

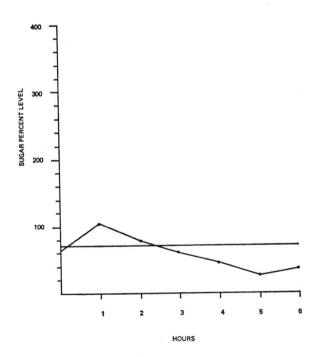

Her physician discussed her case with me, confident that it represented a complete negation of the theory that hypoglycemia may contribute both to asthma and to stomach ulcer, for here was a diabetic whose high blood sugar certainly did not protect her against either of these complicating diseases. I asked for the records of her glucose-tolerance tests only to discover that all had been terminated at the end of the third hour, or earlier. The results of these tests most certainly justified the diagnosis of diabetes. A six-hour test was proposed. See the graph below.

The reader will note that the first three hours of the test are a clear record of diabetic blood sugar levels, but that, just as plainly, the next three hours show a trend toward the hypoglycemia that truly develops in the last hour, with a drop of nearly 40 milligrams percent below the original fasting blood sugar level.

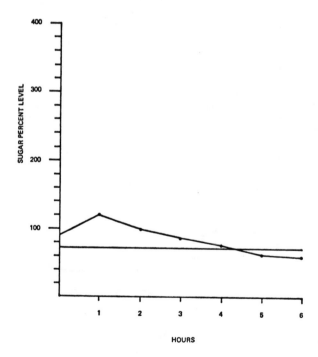

This, of course, is no proof that hypoglycemia was responsible for her asthma and her stomach ulcer. It does prove that a diabetic may suffer both from high blood sugar and low blood sugar at different stages of the response to an oral dose of sugar. Therefore, a diabetic could be susceptible to disorders that are supposed to be prevented by his elevated blood sugar.

The proof of the relationship between the hypoglycemia and the asthma and stomach ulcer came when the woman was placed on a strict hypoglycemia diet. One resembling it, of course, had been prescribed for her ulcer, but that contained some sugar, had been used only at intervals, and was never in use for more than a week at a time. Her dietetic problem was complicated, for previously the amount of carbohydrate in her diet had been linked with her insulin dosage. Now the sugar was entirely eliminated, complex starches substituted, and the overall consumption of carbohydrates reduced. Three years later, she was still receiving the benefits she had derived in the first six months of the hypoglycemia diet. Her asthma had vanished; her stomach ulcer attacks were now rare and could easily be traced to triggering emotional stress; and her diabetes was less severe and under excellent control.

The lesson learned here is that a three-hour glucose-tolerance test may easily identify a diabetic and completely miss a hypoglycemic. The six-hour test is mandatory. Second, hypoglycemia may be related both to asthma and to peptic ulcer. Third, there is obviously something very wrong with the thinking in the medical texts that would label this woman's blood sugar in the sixth hour as *normal*. There *is* a qualifying phrase added to that statement in some texts: "normal, if not accompanied by symptoms of hypoglycemia." But that is not valid, for asthma and peptic ulcer are not regarded by these texts as symptoms of low blood sugar!

The next history reflects most tragically a missed diagnosis of hypoglycemia, with the error compounded by a half-dozen erroneous interpretations of the patient's condition. The subject was an elevator operator, a young man, the father of two children, who suddenly developed a claustrophobia. This, naturally, made his work in the elevator cage unbearable. The anxiety that followed and persisted was blamed on the same conflict which was supposed to be the subconscious basis for the fear of small rooms and crowded places, though one psychiatrist did grant that a claustrophobic working in an elevator might understandably develop an anxiety.

Two blackouts brought him to a clinic, where, although the tracings of the brain waves were normal, he was told that he had a form of epilepsy. This would, of course, make it inadvisable for him to continue a type of work in which the safety of the public is involved. The patient became apprehensive even about walking on the street, and he remained at home while his wife took a job as a domestic. Withdrawing within the home and within himself, he now showed some signs of mildly paranoid behavior—delusions of persecution. This was ascribed to latent homosexuality, a diagnosis with which his wife, in whom he had shown no evidence of sexual interest since his illness began, agreed.

One psychiatrist who saw this man at a clinic had an uneasy conviction that the mental and emotional storms and the "epileptic" blackouts were actually caused by an underlying organic condition, and so it was that, after three years of suffering, the patient was finally subjected to a really complete physical examination that included a three-hour glucose-tolerance test. The response to a dose of sugar was so markedly abnormal that the test was repeated and extended to six hours. The results are on the chart on the next page. The reader will see that the fasting blood sugar level is in itself suspiciously low: the rise after the dose of sugar is abnormally low, indicating either poor absorption, or excessive production of insulin; and, at the fifth hour, the curve dips to a severe hypoglycemic level. The subsequent slight rise, an hour later, may logically be attributed to the effort of the adrenal glands to compensate for the hyperinsulinism by extracting stored sugar (glycogen) from the liver to replenish the blood supply. It is this adrenal effect that is responsible for the feelings of anxiety which in hypoglycemics are then misinterpreted as the product of subconscious conflicts not recognized by the patient.

On a hypoglycemic diet, the patient completely recovered. He learned well the lesson that skipping breakfasts, drinking four to five bottles of cola beverages daily, munching on candy bars, using coffee as others use water, may not only make an invalid—psychiatric and medical—of a normal person, but can threaten the stability of a good marriage.

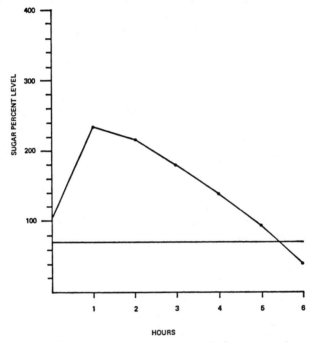

HOURS

A graph of the glucose-tolerance test of the next subject is not necessary. It differs from the preceeding one only in that the final blood sugar level was lower—about 28. Yet the patient's troubles were in some aspects very different. She was a young married woman who at the age of twenty-two gave birth to her baby and subsequently went into what the physician labels "postpartum depression," or what the public calls childbirth insanity. The term is too severe, for in many such cases the emotional disturbances that develop after pregnancy are more like those of a neurosis; but our young woman really seemed psychotic. She did not remember having her baby, and she refused to care for the child. She was unable to do her housekeeping and complained bitterly of claustrophobia, which made it impossible for her to shop for food, and of such sensitivity to noises that the ringing of the telephone sent her into hysteria. Her attention span grew progressively shorter, and she had uncontrollable outbursts of unprovoked tears interspersed with outbursts of maniacal rage. When she discovered that her husband—to whom she had denied sexual relations—had formed a liaison with an attractive neighbor, she attempted to attack him with a knife, and culminated the episode by swallowing a handful of sleeping tablets.

It was at this point that her husband determined to follow the advice he had received from the several psychiatrists he had consulted. The consensus was that he should wait to see if the condition would spontaneously subside. If it did not, shock therapy was recommended, a proposal he bitterly resisted.

The distraught husband had been reading every scrap of medical and psychiatric literature he could find, and by pure and most happy chance, it was at this moment that he heard a broadcast in which the author of this book discussed hypoglycemia. The possibility of this being the problem excited the husband's hopes, but he found it impossible to persuade any of the numerous physicians acquainted with the young woman's condition to order a glucose-tolerance test. In desperation, he took his wife to a medical nutritionist who agreed to administer the test, and the presence of a really severe hypoglycemia was confirmed. The nutritionist's comment is revealing: "I'm not at all startled by the symptoms the low blood sugar caused," he remarked, "but I don't understand how she navigated—how she remained on her feet—and how she escaped brain damage."

On massive doses of liver concentrate and other B Complex supplements in addition to the hypoglycemia diet, she made a reasonably quick and complete recovery. If she sins dietetically, there is a quick exacerbation of some of her old troubles, a reminder that hypoglycemia is really not cured; it is arrested, and the organism prone to low blood sugar never loses the tendency. The interesting feature of this history is the level of her fasting blood sugar and the level at the end of a six-hour test, which to this day remain subnormal even though her symptoms are gone. A nondrinker of milk, she must not only stay with the hypoglycemia diet to remain healthy, but must take calcium supplements, for despite the stability of the blood calcium levels in most individuals, regardless of their diets, it is changeable in many hypoglycemics, and deficiency in ionized blood serum calcium undoubtedly contributes to their tendency to irritability and to muscle spasm.

The lesson learned from this history is that for this young woman, pregnancy was the trigger for hypoglycemia. Stress, which may be anything from prolonged emotional tension to an accident or surgery or pregnancy, is very frequently the prelude to the development of low blood sugar. The secondary stresses alone—excessive use of sugar, excessive caffeine intake, poor nutrition, missed meals—are enough to initiate hypoglycemia in some individuals; others will survive such minor insults without penalty until a major stress is superimposed.

The next "patient" history can be summed up in the phrase "the tired businessman," whose numbers are like the grains of sand on the beach. In this case, we are dealing with the "flat glucose-tolerance curve," which the reader will note is only relatively flat, as shown in the graph on the next page. The blood sugar does not go high enough to nourish brain and nervous system, yet it does not fall low enough, at the end of the test, to be labeled "hypoglycemic," or even "prehypoglycemic"; hence the term "flat."

In this graph, the dotted line indicates the blood sugar levels in average individuals given a dose of sugar; the solid line is the "flat" curve, reflecting the so-called emotional sit-down strike.

The story of the man whose flat curve you have just examined is one that should be considered carefully by business management. The subject was an executive of a large company that had achieved a dominating position in a highly competitive field, with concomitant pressures upon its top and junior executives. This young man had risen to a vice-presidency at the age of thirty-six but found himself, as he later put it, treading a revolving wheel like a caged squirrel, running madly to stay in one place, his company's policy being simple and ruthless: either you earned promotion or you were discarded; no one could stand still.

He found himself more tired on awaking than when he went to bed, and the fatigue increased through the day, with some relief after dinner. When he returned to his home, a short walk from the factory, he slumped into a chair, too tired to be interested in the evening paper, and consumed several cocktails before dinner. His wife, as jaded and weary as he, learned that she could not communicate with him until dinner was over, and conversation then was monosyllabic. She felt completely frustrated by the change in his personality and by the constricted circle in which they existed. The protocol of social relationships in the executive ranks precluded their associating with the lesser executives, dictated their choice of activities and friendships, and limited their selection of a country club, vacation spots, schools for the children, and even the price class of the two cars they owned. The wife found herself at the end of the day filled with the little resentments and hostilities that accrue from a monotonous and repetitive regime of housekeeping, problems with domestic help, normal difficulties with growing children, irritations with neighbors too important to ignore. The husband found himself without ambition, without zest, without the sense of challenge of the kind he had felt when he first began to climb the executive ladder.

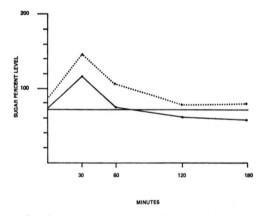

Realizing the discrepancy between the careful maintenance the factory machines received and the physical abuse and mental stress upon executive body and mind, the subject had several times sought a medical explanation of his conversion into the proverbial tired businessman, the result always being "examination essentially negative," usually followed by advice to take more frequent vacations.

He finally developed symptoms that alarmed him—a tightening across his chest, with pain radiating from the left side and down his left arm. He came close at this point to making himself a "cardiac neurotic," like other men who have lost, as he had, a number of male relatives with coronary thrombosis. Aware that a normal electrocardiogram does not preclude a fatal heart attack, he was not reassured by the clean bill of health he was given after several "complete" physical examinations.

The incident that drove him into psychiatric care was a sensation that his head was not attached to his body, a feeling that he was not quite in touch with reality and that his feet, as he put it, were about two inches off the floor. These episodes were followed by severe perspiring and weakness in his legs, which forced him to rest. The brief walk to the factory often brought on these symptoms, worsened the chest pain, and gave him a sense of being short of breath.

Since his physical condition had been exonerated, he now took the company doctor's advice to visit a psychiatrist, who pointed out that what he was describing was the "tired businessman's syndrome" and that it wasn't accidental that his symptoms and his wife's developed at about the same time. (The couple, noting the coincidence, had decided that they both had picked up the chronic, low-grade virus infection with which one of their children had intermittently been battling.)

Psychotherapy did produce some improvement—about 20 percent, the executive thought—but he felt it might have been more effective if his wife had participated. About the time when their marriage seemed to be cracking open from internal pressures, one of the patient's business friends, who himself had been identified as a hypoglycemic, suggested that he, too, undergo a glucose-tolerance test, the result of which you have already examined. The dynamics of the flat sugar-tolerance curve have already been described for the reader. Here we see how lack of challenge and lack of zest produce a disturbance in carbohydrate metabolism, which in turn flattens the body's responses to emotional stimuli, the vicious circle so often involved in hypoglycemic phenomena.

The executive's wife proved as resistant to taking a glucose-tolerance test as she had been to joining him in psychotherapy and was no more cooperative in revising their menus until she yielded to a stern lecture by the physician and read some of the clinical reports on hypoglycemia he supplied and interpreted for her. When she identified many of her husband's symptoms in the case histories of Portis and others working in this field, she finally agreed to cooperate. Her glucose-tolerance curve displayed a moderately severe hypoglycemia.

In this history, it is evident that the hypoglycemia diet not only saved the career of a rising young executive, but quite possibly rescued a marriage as well. We learn from it that there is indeed a vicious circle of zestlessness linked to a flat glucose-tolerance curve, which in turn yields a flat response to emotional stimuli. It matters not at what point you break a vicious circle. Psychotherapy helped; the diet helped more; the two healing modalities produced enough benefit for the patient for him to recapture the meaning of "a man's reach should exceed his grasp, or what's a heaven for?"

Psychiatrists are sometimes exasperated when other schools of medicine fail, as they see it, to give sufficient weight to the emotional dynamics that operate in the sick man; medical practitioners aware of the polymorphic impacts of hypoglycemia on the nervous system and brain are equally intolerant of their colleagues in psychology. The following record compounds these errors and adds another that is, unfortunately, common in medical thinking of today: complete obliviousness to the impact of modern overprocessed carbohydrates on those who constitutionally can not tolerate them.

The patient was forty years of age at the time of this book's first writing. She married at sixteen, wedding the first and only boy, a year older than she, whom she had ever known. She came to marriage armed with all the domestic science she had gleaned from a one-year high school course and applied these skills intensively to her responsibilities as a housekeeper and a cook. Both she and her husband breakfasted on black coffee and cigarettes and both lunched on a skimpy sandwich and a cola drink or two. Dinner was a pizza or a bowl of spaghetti with a couple of meatballs, followed by a piece of commercially baked apple pie, often eaten with ice cream. Macaroni with a small amount of cheese, once in a while a small steak or a pair of slender chops or a piece of fish or chicken—these were their dinner menus. Neither liked vegetables, and both were only mildly tolerant of salads. A quart of milk in their household carried them for three or four days, but the cookie bin needed constant refilling, and their bills for candy, cola drinks, and ice cream were high.

Such was the dietetic preparation for motherhood. A baby was born when the mother was twenty-one and was clearly a victim of her prenatal neglect, for the child was under constant pediatric care for a series of medical problems. For the woman herself, morning sickness was so intense in the first five months of the pregnancy—lasting, indeed, for most of the day—that there were points at which her obstetrician suggested terminating the pregnancy to protect the mother. A week after her return from the maternity hospital, she showed signs of disorientation. She became hysterical without provocation, wept without cause, endured horrible nightmares from which she awoke saturated with perspiration and feeling as if she could not breathe. Her physician tried to wrestle with her sensation that her throat was blocked (globus hystericus—an imaginary ball in the throat), and referred her to a psychiatrist. He treated her on the basis of a postpartum psychosis (insanity after childbirth), for by this time, she clearly had withdrawn from reality, refusing to recognize her baby as her own. Under psychiatric treatment, she began to care for the child, but was so negligent that both her mother and her mother-in-law had to act as substitute mothers. The patient grew more and more claustrophobic, until she refused to use the elevator in her apartment house, could not go to the small laundry room in the basement, and was unable to shop in the crowded supermarkets.

A nutritionist suggested to her physician that many of her symptoms could easily be derived from malnutrition, with the stress and demands of pregnancy superimposed. This was indignantly rejected as food faddism. After all, are not Americans the best-fed people in the world? An added suggestion that a sugar-tolerance test might be revealing, in the context of her exorbitant intake of sugar, was dismissed on similar grounds. Had not Alvarez, of the Mayo Clinic, said that he had not seen a case of hypoglycemia, save the type caused by a tumor, in some thirty years of practice?

Among the troubles that followed her pregnancy, there came a series of cysts of the breasts (cystic mastitis), for which surgery was proposed.

Seeking to escape this treatment, the patient went to a gynecologist, selected because she had heard that he treated these cysts by non-surgical means. This was accurate, for the therapy he was using was purely dietetic, seeking to establish control of hormone overactivity, which he held responsible for the cysts, by encouraging liver degradation of the hormone through the use of a high-vitamin, high-protein, low-carbohydrate diet. Since this treatment has been long known to gynecologists, but employed by perhaps one in a thousand, it is obvious that the long arm of coincidence had reached out to protect this distraught young woman, for is not the diet procedure described basically the same as that used for low blood sugar?

The cysts gradually yielded to the dietetic treatment, and the young woman promptly returned to her old food habits. It was only then that she and her husband realized in retrospect to what an extent better nutrition had improved her "psychotic" behavior, for those symptoms promptly worsened as she reverted to her high intake of processed carbohydrates. She mentioned this observation to the gynecologist, who suggested a glucose-tolerance test, from which she emerged with a diagnosis of severe hypoglycemia, beginning with a fasting blood sugar level of 54 and terminating at the fifth hour with a reading of 42! (Actually, her symptoms became so aggravated that the test could not be continued for the planned six-hour duration.)

The postpartum psychosis is now but an unpleasant and faint memory for this patient and her husband, but her history teaches us that we have yet to achieve a full understanding of the dynamics of disturbed sugar metabolism, for her blood sugar levels to this very day remain abnormally low. Yet she is symptom-free as long as she does not revert to the cookie-cola-candy pattern of biological insult. One of the patient's remarks, in this context, is most interesting: "I remember the posters in my home economics classroom telling us that the calories from sugar are important, and that we need sugar for energy. Why doesn't somebody do something about that?"

Very often, the link between the patient's symptoms and his emotional problems is so very strong and apparent that the psychotherapist will obstinately refuse to entertain any other diagnosis. This was the patent error with a forty-five-year-old married woman who was under psychotherapy for symptoms that had developed as her marriage began to disintegrate and that grew steadily worse after the couple had separated. Her physical complaints began with migraine headaches, gastric cramps, and diarrhea and included chronic fatigue and occasional acute attacks of weakness. She became pathologically apathetic, finally attempting to withdraw entirely from social activities. The critical point was reached the day she finally lost all hope of solving her marital problems. Several years of psychoanalysis were not only unfruitful, but appeared to worsen her physical and emotional complaints.

An interested physician, friendly with the patient, insisted on a glucose-tolerance test, which produced a flat curve. The fasting blood sugar was 90; an hour later, it was 110—less than 50 percent above the starting level, which by the Goodman standard indicates hypoglycemia; she dropped back to 90 at the end of the test. Her symptoms largely disappeared when she was treated for hypoglycemia, and the interesting observation here is the *normal* (by textbook standards) fasting blood sugar level—90! This is at the upper end of the "normal range" and serves to remind us that a single blood sugar level determination can be most misleading.

There are three symptoms that make the experienced practitioner suspicious of hypoglycemia. They include anxiety, compulsive eating—including night raids on the refrigerator—and change of personality. Needless to say, these very symptoms, appraised by the practitioner in psychology, will justify a diagnosis of deep emotional disturbance, at the very least. All three of the symptoms were troubling a young physician, whose anxiety and fears began after he entered private practice. Acute weakness and a feeling of light-headedness followed, particularly two or three hours after a meal. The young medico had to withdraw from his practice, his attacks of weakness and unprovoked phobias severely interfering with his work. The interesting aspect of this record is that the young doctor had already been recognized as a person with functional hypoglycemia; yet he was under psychiatric care and not being treated for his low blood sugar. The fasting blood sugar here, too, was well up at the upper end of the *normal* range—90—and rose to less than 100 at the thirty-minute mark, a typical flat curve, reminding us that the significance of glucose testing lies in the dynamics of the management of sugar by the body. Just as a physician, interpreting a fasting blood sugar level of 90, has no right to assume that the patient is not diabetic, so has he no justification in assuming that he is not hypoglycemic!

As the physician is not immune to low blood sugar, so is the psychologist himself susceptible. The subject of this history is a practitioner who is largely unknown to the public, but so well known and highly regarded among psychologists and psychiatrists that, though the history needs the telling, every effort has been made, by slight changes of the circumstances surrounding the person and his associations, to disguise his identity.

I took his course in advanced social psychology at a major university and observed that the professor, as the long afternoon session proceeded, became progressively paler, seemed to have difficulty with concentration and memory span, and made gestures that were oddly unrelated to the emotional tone of the topics being discussed. Because these symptoms became, to the practiced eye, more pronounced as class and professor reached the point in the afternoon of the *normal* drop in blood sugar, some three hours after lunch, the student was finally induced to broach, hesitantly, the topic to the educator.

He grew even more pale, seemed on the point of fainting, and asked in obvious fright: "Is it noticeable to everybody?" Assured that only the practiced eye made the observation possible, the professor invited his student to discuss the matter in the university cafeteria, where, it should be recorded, his snack selection was a sugar-coated Danish pastry and a cola drink. "I have thought of suicide," he confessed (while ingesting some eleven teaspoonfuls of sugar in his pastry and beverage). "The feeling of detachment from reality, as though my head were not in touch with my body, was—I diagnosed it—a certain sign of a beginning psychosis, particularly with my nightmares, troubles in concentrating, and the disintegration of what used to be a photographic memory. So I planned to fall under a truck because I wanted it to look like an accident." Asked why a suicide would need such a facade, he said: "I am too well known in the field of psychology. After all, I helped to develop concepts that radically reshaped many of the approaches to problems in my particular field of specialization. I felt that my going psychotic—or alcoholic, for that matter—would give psychology an undeserved black eye."

The mention of alcoholism brought more questions. Yes, he had been drinking secretively because it seemed at least temporarily to relieve some of his symptoms. He confessed to alternating between the bottle and the candy jar, sucking on hard candies whenever he had the opportunity. There was—as he termed it, in typical psychological jargon—free-floating anxiety, an unexplained and unprovoked sensation of imminent disaster, which attached itself to any event, logically or not.

The professor was referred to an internist for a glucose-tolerance test. It revealed a severe hypoglycemia. Treatment was instituted, and response was prompt. A brilliant mind was restored to full function, a fine educator and practitioner to full efficiency. While he gave at least lip service to remaining on the hypoglycemia diet, he confessed that he found it difficult to abstain entirely from alcoholic beverages. He was warned that this was a path to relapse and, indeed, to chronic alcoholism. At this point, however, his marriage, which had been under constant stress during his period of hypoglycemic symptoms, collapsed. The psychologist began to drink again, left the diet, and all symptoms returned and intensified. He became a full-fledged alcoholic, managing to continue to practice and to teach only because his drinking was secretive and confined to the privacy of his home. The patient himself agrees with his physician that if he had continued the hypoglycemia diet, he would today be a well man, free of compulsive drinking and the symptoms that he had interpreted as pre-psychotic.

The lesson we learn from this case is found in the (completely erroneous) diagnosis of the psychologist, which had been given to him by a fellow practitioner. In part, it read: "Despite the patient's accomplishments in clinical and social psychology, he has a deep-seated sense of insecurity which will not permit him to relax, and which has thereby denied him a vacation for more than ten years. His sensation of detachment from reality reflects a very real need to escape it . . ." and so on. The incident brings to mind a suggestion made by a physician who was wary of the possible cancer-producing effects of estrogenic hormones and proposed that patients might be less haphazardly dosed with these substances if each label were required by law to carry the legend: "Doctor—are you sure your patient is not cancer-prone, does not have cancer?" By the same token, the history of the psychologist suggests that in every psychological case record, each page should carry the legend: "The psyche is housed in the soma!"

# 9. The Diets for Hypoglycemia

Note the plural: diets for hypoglycemia. There is no such entity as a single diet for a single disorder. Disorders have different impacts and different causes and thus different treatments. Even identical twins may differ biochemically, and thereby in nutritional needs and tolerances, and if that is true for healthy twins, it is triply so for the sick. You are a unique biochemical event, with no exact duplicate among the billions of human beings. For this reason, observe the following:

1. Keep away from books that offer a single system of diet—for whatever purpose—for all readers. They have to be wrong for some people, and you might be one of the victims of generalizations in a field that doesn't allow for them.

2. And, as the preceding warning also implies, stay away from those—lay or professional—who prescribe a uniform diet for hypoglycemia. There are those who insist that high complex carbohydrates are the way to go, and that high protein or fat are passports to nothing but trouble. There are also those who, conversely, warn readers that high-protein diets cause "dire troubles," to quote an ignorant physician, and who seem blind to the fact that hypoglycemics usually arrive at their troubles not by overeating protein, but by stuffing themselves with sugars and starches. The safe conclusion, arrived at by working with thousands of hypoglycemics, is that it is best to start with adequate protein intake, a normal fat quota in part derived from a modest amount of vegetable oils, and a limited carbohydrate intake, in the complex form, using the glycemic index to avoid those that act like simple sugars. Experience will then teach whether a given hypoglycemic does well with this dietary plan or needs a drop or an elevation in complex carbohydrate levels. Sometimes as little as 20 grams of carbohydrate, up or down, will prove to be the critical difference.

This book therefore presents two diets, the first more liberal with carbohydrates, and the second limiting intake of complex starches to approximately 60 grams daily. For the first, I drew upon the experience of my longtime collaborator, Herman Goodman, MD. The second diet, less liberal in carbohydrate, is mine. We see eye to eye on the need for reduction of sugar intake as an aid to better health, as a help in preventing hypoglycemia, as a sine qua non in treating it. We are as one on the need in this disorder for supplementing the diet with protein and Vitamin B Complex to help to restore proper function of the liver, which we see as a critical factor (and a neglected one) in regulation of blood sugar levels. But when we approach the diet itself, physician and nutritionist part company—however amicably. The medical man gives short shrift to those who complain about the acrid taste of needed medicines and is equally impatient with those who find a prescribed diet to be distasteful, bland, monotonous, and unpalatable. The nutritionist, who remembers that people have chosen starvation rather than consume unfamiliar or disliked foods,* tends to keep a stricter eye on the eye-and-palate appeals of recipes and menus.

And so it is that two diets for hypoglycemia are presented, alike in restriction of sugar intake and in emphasis on protein and fat intake, but differing, for reasons stated, in allowances of the complex starches. One of these, obviously, will be a more palatable diet, achieved at the expense of more hours spent in the kitchen. Yours is the choice, but I suggest that you remember that this information is offered to help you to cooperate with your own physician, as the person who best knows you and is best qualified thereby to guide and appraise your progress. He will be needed, too, for prescription of certain medications that some patients will need to accelerate their recovery from low blood sugar.

Dr. Herman Goodman has found the following dietary recommendations to be effective in the control of functional hypoglycemia:

1. Eat as much as you wish at each meal and between meals, choosing only from the permitted foods. Let your scale tell you when portions (rather than frequency of eating) must be reduced. If you are overweight, it is easily possible to lose weight while still controlling low blood sugar. If you are underweight, be of good cheer, for many who

---

* When pernicious anemia was a sentence to slow death, and liver, three times daily, was shown to halt the degeneration of nervous system and brain, patients vowed that they would choose death rather than eat liver thrice daily!

could not gain while suffering from hypoglycemia, promptly did so when the disorder was brought under control.

2. Choose from: LEAN MEAT, FISH, POULTRY: broiled, baked, or roasted. Boiling is less satisfactory for retention of nutrients. Avoid fried food. Eat fish at least five times each week. Use other protein sources, such as pressed cottage cheese, which is sold as farmer cheese and pot cheese. VEGETABLES: Spinach, chard, broccoli, kale, cabbage, cauliflower, string beans, squash, eggplant, asparagus, lettuce, tomato, cucumber. FRUIT: Apples, pears, peaches, melons, berries—fresh or water-packed canned. Eat oranges and grapefruit in moderation. Avoid candied dried fruit. BEVERAGES: Water, weak tea, Sanka or Decaf (percolated type), skim milk, unsweetened fruit juice.

3. Do not eat starchy foods (except allowed bread), sugar and foods made with sugar—such as candy, cake, pie, cookies, chewing gum— crackers, matzohs, pizza, Chinese sweet and pungent dishes, sauces, gravies, dressings made with flour, ketchup, and canned foods packed with sugar.

4. Do not drink alcoholic beverages, regular coffee or strong tea, chocolate, cocoa, cola beverages, conventional (sugared) soft drinks, other drinks made with sugar, corn syrup, glucose, etc. Do not abuse beverages made with synthetic sweeteners. *

5. Weigh yourself each morning at the same time. Consult your physician to decide your ideal weight. Reach it and stay there! Don't forget that the high-sugar diet, which predisposes us to low blood sugar, with its corollary craving for sweets, is often the reason for obesity. You *can* find the way back to slimness.

*Outline for the Day with Suggested Time and Edibles*

BEFORE BREAKFAST: Use your blender or beater to mix one teaspoonful each of dry skim milk powder, protein powder, glycine, and primary food brewer's yeast powder. Liquefy in water, unsweetened fruit juice,

---

* I believe that in hypersensitive individuals, the sweet taste of synthetic sweeteners may touch off the pancreas by a kind of conditioned reflex action. If this sounds preposterous, remember that the gallbladder in sensitive persons has been seen to contract when its owner scented food being fried.

or fluid skim milk. Add any flavoring, such as real vanilla, that pleases you. Never miss this supplement; it is a critical part of the dietetic procedure.

BREAKFAST: Fruit, from list above. Two slices of ham or bacon (remove as much fat as possible), broiled to render lower in fat (bacon should be brittle). A substitute for ham or bacon is hoop cheese, which is pot cheese in the form used by bakers for making cheese cake. (Farmer cheese in foil packages is to be avoided.) One thin slice of bread or toast, with butter. Water, weak tea, Sanka, Decaf, with skim milk. No sugar.

TWO HOURS LATER: Farmer, pot, imported Swiss or cheddar cheese. Water, weak tea, or skim milk.

LUNCH: Fair-sized portion of lean meat, fish, poultry, lean meat hamburger, or half cup of drained canned salmon, sardines, or tunafish.

TWO HOURS AFTER LUNCH: Repeat midmorning snack.

EVENING MEAL: Fruit or juice from list. Lean meat, etc., as at lunch, with vegetables chosen from list. No substitutions. Allowed beverage.

BEFORE RETIRING: Fruit from approved list, and piece of cheese.

Avoid tobacco. M. G. Berry, MD, in 1959 wrote a paper describing a group suffering from emotional instability, apprehension, and insecurity. The glucose-tolerance tests reported showed results identical with or at least similar to those obtained in functional hypoglycemia. Yet the patients—all heavy smokers—did not respond to the low blood sugar diet. The only help for this type of low blood sugar—tobacco hypoglycemia—is a total halt in smoking.

A further word of advice: let the islets of Langerhans (source of insulin in the pancreas) forget to react violently to carbohydrate. Visualize the islets as sleeping, and don't awaken them by cheating with even the smallest amount of sugar at any time. Watch your Sundays: brunch is not an excuse for committing gastronomic suicide with carbohydrates.

## The Diet For All Those Who Are Hypoglycemic, and For Those Who Combine Overweight or Underweight With Low Blood Sugar, With A Few Concessions To Hypoglycemic Gourmets

By way of proving that calorie intake is not the entire explanation of weight gain, there are those with low blood sugar who—though saturated with the cakes and candies they crave—are markedly underweight. Others are overweight, and the majority, probably, hover around normal weight levels. The nutritionist's diets for hypoglycemia are tailored to the obese. Those whose weight is normal can ignore the careful sizing of portions in the menus, and those who are underweight should increase the sizes of portions. Both groups, of course, will observe carefully the restrictions on intake of sugar and starch and, in changing the amounts of proteins and fats, will preserve the proportions outlined in the following plan, so that dietary balances are preserved.

If you are obese, you will be startled by the amount of weight that will slip away in a few weeks on this diet, despite a generous and satisfying amount of food. Plateaus will be encountered when loss of weight will slow or stop, but the course will, if you persevere, resume downward. *

It may seem paradoxical that restricting your intake of carbohydrates will, if you are underweight, often help weight gain. After all, when you indulged your sweet tooth, it didn't help you to put on pounds, did it? More of the complex starches are allowed when weight gain is too slow or when the hypoglycemic appears to need more of them.

An observation of interest to both the lean and the fat: restriction of the intake of processed starches and sugars and limitation of total sugar and starch intake have a curious result in that weight gain and weight

---

* In cases of metabolic obesity associated with hypoglycemia, two procedures may be helpful. One is elimination of allergenic foods from your diet, and the second, to repeat an important suggestion, is the use of edible-grade linseed oil, a tablespoonful daily, as a supplement to the vegetable oil already mentioned. In some cases of metabolic obesity, where ordinary reducing diets have little or no effect, the use of the oil with a low-carbohydrate diet may cause sporadic but satisfying losses of weight—as much as fifteen pounds in a weekend.

loss are more likely to be achieved in the parts of the body where they are needed. It is a kind of biochemical spot reduction for the overweight, with the loss of dimension completely out of proportion to the loss in pounds. For the underweight, the converse change takes place, and it is often similarly dramatic. The normal in weight who have fat in the wrong places may be pleasantly astonished to find those difficult areas shrinking, even without weight loss. Lecithin or a supplement of choline, inositol, and methionine, available in health-food stores, may help fat redistribution.

The sizes of portions specified in the following menus, then, are to be observed strictly only by the overweight.

Begin the day with the pre-breakfast drink previously recommended: one teaspoonful each of dry skim milk powder, protein powder, glycine, and brewer's yeast. (Choose a yeast high in protein and Vitamin B Complex, and be sure it's soluble. Do not accept torula yeast.) These ingredients can be blended with unsweetened fruit juice or fluid skim milk, Add flavoring, such as real vanilla, to taste. *

Use as you please, within reasonable bounds:

Salt substitute
Sugar substitutes (saccharin)—except during first five months of
    pregnancy
Clear broth (not bouillon cubes)
Unsweetened whole gelatin
Lemon
Vinegar
All spices, save celery salt and garlic salt
All herbs
Sugar-free soft drinks (not cola type)—not more than 8 ounces
    daily
Coffee free of caffeine (Sanka, Decaf)
Desserts from approved ones mentioned later

---

* If previous eating habits have been poor, as in most hypoglycemics, it is well to add a multiple vitamin, multiple mineral, and liver supplement to this regime. Raw liver is available in tablet form.

Avoid like the plague:

Margarine
Sugar-sweetened soft drinks
Sugar-sweetened juices, canned, and frozen fruits
Vegetables packed in sugar-sweetened liquid or sauce (You must
    read labels carefully!)
Sugar (regardless of its color)
Molasses
Honey
Cookies, cakes, crackers, pretzels, popcorn, potato chips, and all
    starch-sugar snack foods.

The most important rule is to eat six meals per day, with a protein food (eggs, meat, fish, fowl, or dairy products such as cheese) of animal origin in each meal. Select the protein foods from the list that follows.

Each day, eat one egg, cooking method of your choice. If fried, use Teflon type of pan and no fat. It is wisest to include the egg in your daily menu, but if you choose, you can substitute an extra two ounces of meat for it.

Eat 11 ounces daily of meat, fish, and poultry. This is the cooked weight. Make it 13 ounces if you omit egg. Don't cheat yourself—a boneless fillet of beef that weighs 4 ounces, uncooked, will weigh 3 ounces when cooked. A chop that weighs 5 ounces raw, will yield about 3 ounces cooked.

If you want to make a substitution for the meat, an ounce of meat can be replaced by one-fourth cup of cottage cheese. Two ounces of meat may be replaced by an ounce of American, cheddar, or similarly highly fermented cheese. Occasionally, which means no more than twice weekly, an ounce of meat may be replaced by one tablespoonful of peanut butter. Choose the brand that is less sweet, or if available, buy peanut butter freshly prepared, without additives and sugar. A little orange juice will render it less "tacky" and it is a surprisingly palatable addition.

The preferred type of salad oil to use is sesame or safflower. These are sources of needed unsaturated fat which, if purchased in health-food stores, will not contain BHT and BHA, objectionable preservatives.

Keep the oil in a sealed container in the refrigerator, for oxidized (rancid) oil is harmful. Use Vitamin E (in the form of mixed tocopherols) as a supplement, to perform the same service within the body: keeping the oil from oxidizing.

A maximum of 5 teaspoonfuls of oil is the daily ration, both for cooking and as a salad dressing. Additional oil, in the form of edible-grade linseed oil, may be helpful in resistant obesity. (see footnote, page 155). While mayonnaise is palatable, it is often a vehicle both for undesirable additives and for partially hydrogenated fats, which are dangerous. If you wish to use commercial salad dressings, choose the brands that are free of both ingredients. Usually these are available refrigerated, cold being a good substitute for other preservatives.

Two cups daily is the permitted amount of skim milk or partially defatted buttermilk. You should eat two servings of fruit daily, chosen from the types and in the amounts in the following list:

| FRUITS | AMOUNT IN ONE SERVING |
|---|---|
| Apple | 1 small (2-inch diameter) |
| Applesauce | ½ cup (no added sugar) |
| Apricots, fresh | 2 medium |
| Apricots, dried | 4 halves |
| Banana | ½ small |
| Blackberries | 1 cup |
| Blueberries | ⅔ cup |
| Cantaloupe | ¼ (6-inch diameter) |
| Cherries | 10 large |
| Cranberries | 1 cup |
| Dates | 2 |
| Figs, fresh | 2 large |
| Figs, dried | 1 small |
| Grapefruit | ½ small |
| Grapefruit juice | ½ cup |
| Grapes | 12 large |
| Grape juice | ¼ cup |
| Honeydew melon | ⅛ medium |

| Mango | 1 small |
| Nectarine | 1 medium |
| Orange | 1 small |
| Orange juice | ½ cup |
| Papaya | ⅓ medium |
| Peach | 1 medium |
| Pear | 1 small |
| Persimmon | ½ small |
| Pineapple | ½ cup |
| Pineapple juice | ⅓ cup |
| Plums | 2 medium |
| Prunes, dried | 2 medium |
| Raspberries | 1 cup |
| Rhubarb | 1 cup |
| Strawberries | 1 cup |
| Tangerine | 1 cup |
| Watermelon | 1 cup |

Be warned that frozen fruits often yield more calories from sugar than from the fruit itself. Avoid canned fruits packed in syrup, whether light or heavy syrup. Choose the water-packed or artificially sweetened variety.

You *must* consume at least *two* cups of vegetables daily, and you can have as much as *four* cups of vegetables daily, chosen from the following list:

Asparagus
Avocado
Beet greens
Broccoli
Brussels sprouts
Cabbage
Celery
Chard
Chicory
Collards
Cucumbers
Dandelion
Eggplant
Endive
Escarole
Green or wax beans
Green pepper
Kale
Kohlrabi
Leeks
Lettuce
Mushrooms
Mustard
Radishes
Sauerkraut
Spinach
String beans
Summer squash
Tomatoes
Tomato juice
Turnip greens
Watercress

You may have up to one-half slice of bread with each meal and snack. Note, however, that bread made from whole grain—whole wheat, whole rye—is better for you.

Three slices of bread daily may be excessive for some hypoglycemics and for some overweight individuals. More urgent: remember that the starch of bread does not act like starch but more like sugar, being quickly absorbed. A generous spreading of butter may slow the absorption, and the fiber of whole wheat may be helpful, too. Only trial and error can determine one's needs and tolerances for complex carbohydrates, both in terms of weight loss and in terms of hypoglycemia. If wheat triggers hypoglycemia symptoms, which it may in some individuals, a trial of rice (as in rice cakes) is in order. Other substitutions for a half slice of bread would be any of the following vegetables: a half cup of beets, pumpkin, carrots, onions, peas, rutabagas, turnips, or winter squash.

*The Outline of a Meal Pattern Complying with These Requirements*

PRE-BREAKFAST PROTEIN DRINK

BREAKFAST

Fruit or juice
1 egg
1 ounce meat or meat substitute, such as cheese or fish
½ slice whole wheat bread with 1 teaspoon butter
1 cup weak tea, sweetened artificially if desired

MIDMORNING SNACK

1 cup skim milk, flavored, if desired, with vanilla or other sugar-
  free natural flavor
1 ounce meat or meat substitute (see recipes)

LUNCH

3 ounces meat (cooked weight) or meat substitute
1 serving vegetables
1 slice bread with 1 teaspoon butter

Green salad with vegetable oil or mayonnaise (1 teaspoon)
Dessert from approved selection (see recipes)
Weak tea or artificially sweetened soft drink
*Note:* a second vegetable may be selected from the list proposed
as bread substitutes.

### MIDAFTERNOON SNACK
2 ounces meat or meat substitute (see snack recipes)
½ cup skim milk, flavored if desired
½ slice bread with small amount butter

### DINNER
3 ounces meat or meat substitute
Vegetable
Green salad with vegetable oil or mayonnaise dressing
1 serving approved fruit
Approved dessert
Weak tea or other approved beverage

### EVENING SNACK
½ cup skim milk, flavored if desired
1 ounce meat or meat substitute (see snack recipes)

## Suggestions for Between-Meal Snacks

These snacks are all high in protein, though it is possible, of course,
to use up some of the allotted bread intake at these little meals. To keep
low the amount of carbohydrates from bread, one can use brown rice
cakes, which are available in health food stores. These weigh half as
much as slices of bread, and, when pre-warmed, are quite palatable,
satiate the craving for carbohydrates (which will lessen as the low-sugar
diet is followed) at the snacks, and provide a vehicle for the protein
foods.

Note that snack portions are one ounce—for reducers.

COTTAGE CHEESE, a frequent choice of those on the hypoglycemia diet, can be made more palatable by adding chopped dill, chopped chives, chopped onion or scallion, shredded spinach, poppy seeds, caraway seeds, or horseradish.

HAM HORN: Press pot cheese through strainer. Add enough yogurt to make a soft paste and a little chopped dill pickle. Roll this in a paper-thin piece of ham, securing it with a toothpick to make a small horn.

TONGUE–CHEESE HORN: Fill paper-thin tongue slice, rolled into horn shape, with Neufchatel cheese.

DOUGHLESS PIZZA:

   ½ pound lean beef
   ¼ small can tomato paste
   2 fresh tomatoes
   1 medium onion
   1 pinch pepper
   ⅛ teaspoon each of sweet basil, oregano, paprika

Pepper meat, and knead. Line small Pyrex dish with meat as substitute for pizza shell. Chop tomatoes with onions and mix with tomato paste and spices. Fill meat shell with mixture. Add a touch of oregano on top and bake to preferred doneness at 350°.

TUNA IN CUCUMBER: Hollow out ½ cucumber, stuff with 1 ounce tuna fish mixed with 1 teaspoonful salad dressing (see page 158).

CHEESE FOR SNACKS: Cheeses should not be restricted in variety. Use Brie, American, cheddar, pot, farmer, cottage, and be wary only of cheese *spreads*, for these may be diluted with cornstarch or other carbohydrates. Gouda, Swiss, and processed cheeses (Velveeta and others of this type) are all good choices. The cheese, for variety, may be combined with another protein: ham as a blanket for a piece of Gouda is delightful, and good nutrition, too.

CELERY STICK AND POT CHEESE (1 ounce): Press cheese through strainer. Moisten it with a small amount of yogurt, buttermilk, or skim milk. Flavor it with chopped green pepper, watercress, parsley, or pimiento, chopped fine. Fill celery stick with mixture.

SNACK BEVERAGE: Take ½ cup plain yogurt (fruit varieties contain an unbelievable amount of sugar), and fizz it in a tall glass with carbonated water (club soda) or carbonated mineral water.

STUFFED EGG SNACK: Mash hard-cooked yolks of 3 eggs until fine and crumbly. Add 1 ounce melted butter, ⅛ teaspoon salt, dash pepper, ⅛ teaspoon prepared mustard, ½ teaspoon minced onion, ⅙ cup flaked tuna, cut-up shrimp, or crab meat. Mix until smooth, and fill hollows in egg whites, garnishing with slices of olive, pimiento, or parsley. Yields 6 stuffed-egg halves. Reducers should eat only one.

SNACK DESSERT AND BEVERAGE: Pour a little low-calorie ginger ale over 2 tablespoons of nonfat milk powder. Use rest of soda as beverage.

CHEESE–APPLE SNACK: Combine a wedge of Gruyère cheese with ½ small apple.

CHICKEN SNACK: Spread 1 ounce of commercial chicken spread on thin whole wheat cracker.

KOSHER SNACK: Broiled beef fry—1 ounce of beef (smoked beef plate, used instead of bacon in orthodox Jewish diet*). Beverage: V-8 vegetable juice cocktail or equivalent.

YOGURT SNACK: Plain yogurt (4 ounces), with vanilla or almond extract to taste.

COLESLAW SNACK: 1 ounce sliced meat, such as roast beef or tongue, rolled and filled with coleslaw.

SHRIMP SNACK: Commercial frozen shrimp cocktail (1-ounce portion for reducers) is a convenient snack food, very rich in protein. So are canned smoked oysters.

MUSHROOM SNACK: Stuffed mushrooms (2 ounces) filled (topped) with paste made from pot cheese, curry powder, and salt or salt substitute.

PEAR SNACK: Partially scoop out small pear, and fill with 1 ounce soft Camembert cheese.

HAMBURGER: 1 ounce ground chuck, with a touch of garlic, 1 teaspoon tomato juice, and a dash of tarragon. Broil.

These suggestions do not, of course, exhaust the possibilities, but they do emphasize that a low-sugar diet, restricted in starch, does not have to be monotonous and can be attractive even to those who love to eat. Two points must be emphatically repeated: the snacks are *important* (if they are not taken, the appetite for sweets may stir again), and a

---

* The nitrates of frankfurters and other delicatessen foods can cause the body to manufacture nitrosamines, which are potent causes of cancer. Some protection is achieved by taking a supplement of Vitamin C or Vitamin E after such meals.

substantial breakfast, of the type outlined, is mandatory. If you are hypoglycemic *and* overweight, you will be tempted to decide that taking less food, fewer snacks, and a smaller breakfast will help you to reduce more quickly. It won't. The instructions given here have been thoroughly tested and they should be followed implicitly.

To emphasize the point that one can cope with hypoglycemia and still eat enjoyable, attractive meals, here are a few menus, complete with recipes.

### BREAKFAST

½ tangerine, sliced
1 poached egg with 1 ounce of bacon or beef fry
½ slice of whole wheat or whole rye toast with 1 teaspoon
    butter, or ½ portion of oatmeal, small amount skim milk,
    artificial sweetener, 1 teaspoon butter
Weak tea (This need not be conventional tea. Try jasmine tea or
    tea with cinnamon.)

### MIDMORNING SNACK

Ham horn
½ slice whole wheat or whole rye bread
½ cup skim milk

### LUNCH

Mushrooms sautéed with ground meat (3 ounces total)
Grilled tomato
Boston lettuce with scallions, cucumber, oil dressing, and
    seasoning
½ slice whole wheat, whole rye bread, or Finn Crisp with 1
    teaspoon butter
Zabaglione
Weak tea or Sanka (percolated type)

### RECIPES

*Mushrooms Sautéed with Ground Meat*                    (Serves 4)

Piece beef suet, or 3 ounces diced pork lard
¾ pound beef or other lean meat, ground fine
Salt and pepper
1 pound mushrooms, minced
1 tablespoon parsley

Render suet or lard in skillet, and sauté ground meat in fat until brown. After adding mushrooms and parsley, sauté 15 minutes longer, and serve. A 3-ounce portion should be the limit for overweights.

### Grilled Tomato

Lightly dust slices of tomato with oregano, bread with small amount of wheat germ, and grill under medium flame until hot.

### Zabaglione                                                    (Serves 4)

6 eggs, separated
3 tablespoons sherry or Marsala wine
¾ teaspoon liquid saccharin *

Mix wine with saccharin and egg yolks in top of double boiler. Beat constantly as mixture cooks over gently simmering water until thick and light. At serving time, beat egg whites until stiff. Then fold yolk mixture into whites. Serve either warm or chilled in wine glasses.

MIDAFTERNOON SNACK
Brie cheese (1 ounce) on brown rice wafers
Tomato juice (4–6 ounces)

* At the time of revision of this text, the new protein (phenylalanine-aspartane) sweeteners cannot be recommended. Among other allegations, to be proved or disproved, they are said to cause a relentless craving for sugars and starch.

DINNER

Slice of melon with thin slice ham
Pot roast in red wine
Cooked carrots with anise (optional)
¼ head lettuce with Russian dressing
Junket with berries
Weak tea or Sanka

RECIPES

*Pot Roast in Red Wine*                                    (Serves 6–8)

Use 4 pounds inexpensive cut lean beef (chuck) or rolled roast with fat
trimmed. Marinate overnight in:

    1 cup canned beef bouillon
    1½ cups dry red wine
    1 clove garlic, chopped
    2 large onions, sliced
    2 bay leaves
    2 slices lemon
    3 cloves
    ¼ teaspoon oregano
    ¼ teaspoon celery seed
    10 black peppercorns, cracked
    1 teaspoon salt or salt substitute

After marinating meat, brown all sides over low flame and discard
dissolved fat. Add marinade and bring to boil. Then cover and cook in
preheated oven at 450°. If you want really tender pot roast, reduce
temperature to 250° after 10 minutes and cook for 2 to 2½ hours. Put
meat on warm plate and strain liquid into bowl, retaining vegetables. If
fat content is excessive, bring it down by skimming with paper towel.
Slice meat, add gravy, cooked carrots and onions, and serve with
mashed potatoes (not for you, however). Your portion is 3 ounces if
you're overweight.

*Cooked Carrots with Anise*

Prepare carrots in minimum amount of boiling water. Drain and roll them in mint or parsley (finely chopped) or sprinkle them with a few anise seeds. An alternate is a fair amount of tarragon in butter sauce.

*Junket with Berries* (Serves 2)

> 1 junket tablet (Tablets, unlike the powder, are
>    unsweetened.)
> 1 cup double-strength nonfat milk, liquefied (Use ½
>    amount of water specified for reconstituting
>    powdered skim milk.)
> 4 ¼-grain saccharin tablets
> ½ teaspoon pure vanilla extract

Mix ingredients and, stirring constantly for not more than 1 minute, heat to the lukewarm stage—about the temperature desired in a baby formula, or, if you have a cooking thermometer, not over 110°. When warm enough, add junket tablet dissolved in ½ tablespoon cold water. Stir quickly for 10 seconds, pour into cups, let stand 20 minutes, and then refrigerate. Serve with stewed or fresh blackberries or strawberries (6 if you're overweight).

NIGHT SNACK (per serving)
Thin slice chicken, rolled and filled with coleslaw
½ cup skim milk

Here is another day's menu. Do not forget that each day must begin with the pre-breakfast protein drink.

BREAKFAST

1 small orange
Swiss cheese eggs
½ slice toast with 1 teaspoon butter
Weak tea or Sanka

RECIPE

*Swiss Cheese Eggs*                                          (Serves 1)

> 2 eggs
> ⅛ pound Swiss cheese
> ¼ teaspoon pepper
> ¼ teaspoon dry mustard
> Dash of paprika, garlic, cayenne pepper

Grate cheese and separate eggs. Add most of cheese and remaining ingredients to yolks. Beat in the unbeaten whites. Place mixture in Pyrex dish. Top with remainder of grated cheese, and bake slowly until brown on top.

### MIDMORNING SNACK
Shrimp cocktail (1 ounce)
Low-calorie cranberry juice (4 ounces)

### LUNCH
Carrot and celery sticks
Ground meat tarragon (3 ounces)
½ slice bread and butter
Romaine and plum tomato salad with vinegar and oil dressing
1 ring of pineapple, packed in its own juice
Tomato juice with dash of A-1 sauce or equivalent
Weak tea or low-calorie soft drink (not cola!) or Sanka

### MIDAFTERNOON SNACK
Thin slice of smoked salmon with 1 ounce of cheese
Yogurt fizz (½ cup yogurt in tall glass with carbonated water or low-calorie club soda to fill)

### DINNER
V-8 juice (4 ounces)
Chicken, broiled in orange juice
Shoestring eggplant

½ slice bread, or 1 brown rice cake with butter
Pineapple-lime salad
Baked custard
Weak tea, stirred with cinnamon stick

RECIPES

*Chicken in Orange Juice*    (Serves 4)

1 3-pound lean broiling chicken, halved
1 clove garlic, halved
½ teaspoon tarragon
Salt or salt substitute and pepper to taste
½ cup chopped scallions
2 cups orange juice, unstrained

Rub chicken with cut half of garlic clove and mixture of tarragon, salt, and pepper. Place chicken, skin side up, in shallow baking dish, and pour 1 cup juice over chicken. Sprinkle on the scallions. Broil until chicken is brown on each side, adding more juice if needed.

*Shoestring Eggplant*    (Serves 4)

1 small eggplant
1 tablespoon water
1 egg, beaten
½ cup bread crumbs and ½ cup wheat germ
Salt or salt substitute

Pare eggplant, and cut into ½-inch cubes. Soak cubes in cold salted water for ½ hour, and then dry. Dip them into egg to which you have added 1 tablespoon water. Roll them in crumb-wheat germ mixture and fry in about ½ inch of hot cottonseed oil until eggplant is golden brown. Do not let oil reach smoking point. Drain on absorbent paper and salt before serving.

*Pineapple-Lime Salad*                                           (Serves 4)

    1 cup pineapple packed in its own juice (unsweetened)
    1 teaspoon pimiento, chopped
    1 teaspoon diced celery
    Salt or salt substitute, to taste
    1 tablespoon vinegar
    1 envelope artificially sweetened lime gelatin
    ½ cup hot water

Cut pineapple into cubes. Dissolve gelatin in hot water, and when it begins to set, add fruit, celery, and pimientos that have been marinated (2 hours) in vinegar and salt or salt substitute. Let stand in individual molds until set, and serve on crisp lettuce leaf.

*Baked Custard*                                                 (Serves 1)

    ½ cup whole milk
    1 egg
    ⅛ teaspoon almond extract
    Nutmeg

Scald milk. Beat egg slightly. Add scalded milk to egg and mix well. Add almond extract and, if desired, liquid artificial sweetener. Pour into custard cup that has been rinsed in cold water, and bake in 325° oven for 45 minutes. Results are better if custard is baked with cup surrounded by water. When a pointed knife inserted in custard emerges clean, it is done. Do not hesitate to prolong baking time for browning and the doneness you prefer. Vanilla, lemon, or maple may be used instead of almond.

NIGHT SNACK

Strawberry "soda" (4 large strawberries blended with ½ cup of
    skim milk)
1 ounce cottage cheese with garden salad (available commercially)

The point has been made by these menus. No one who likes to cook need complain that the hypoglycemia diet is distasteful. No one who wants to lose weight while controlling hypoglycemia need fear the generous portions allowed in a low-carbohydrate diet. Paradoxically, while vegetable oils are rich in calories, they *are* needed, do not interfere with weight loss, and confer needed nutritional dividends.

## Fiber—the Friend of the Hypoglycemic

Rapid absorption of food is the enemy of the hypoglycemic. The fuel for a hypoglycemic should be like kerosene rather than like gasoline. This explains the thrust of the diet for low blood sugar, which excludes sugar and the highly processed starches which are rapidly absorbed. The body of the hypoglycemic is unable to cope with sudden, large rises in blood sugar or, for that matter, with subsequent large drops in blood sugar. It is as if the hypoglycemic were a person in whom the wisdom of the body has somehow gone awry. The prohibition of high intake of sugar—not only the familiar white crystals in the bowl, but the simple sugars of fruit and the metabolic sources of simple sugars, such as overrefined starches—becomes understandable. Only recently, though, have nutritionists discovered that some of the complex starches act like sugar. A typical example is a baked potato. When it is eaten dry, without the skin, its starch behaves exactly like sugar. If you take the potato with sour cream or butter, it acts like starch, which is to say that the absorption is slowed up by the fat.

Recent studies have indicated that the freedom of some primitive groups from bowel cancer, so frequent in our country, is due to their higher intake of food fiber (a long way of saying that they eat their grains unprocessed). Still more recently, another dividend from a high-fiber diet has been realized. Fiber acts for food generally as the butter acts for the baked potato: it slows its absorption. This suggests that you should not only shift to the whole grains, in place of white flour, white rice, processed cornmeal, processed rye, and buckwheat, but use bran in modest amounts with each meal. (You must be sure, of course, that allergy to wheat is not a problem).

Not only does intake of fiber helpfully slow the absorption of food, but, in many individuals, it is the key to freedom from constipation and the Pandora's box of troubles that accompany a chronic case, including diverticulosis and diverticulitis. The use of bran, however, does require a little expertise. You should not use large quantities initially. Start with a minimal amount and gradually increase it. The optimal quantity—which may be very different from person to person—has been reached when a bowel movement is well formed but soft, evacuation is easy, without straining, and the stool is virtually odorless.

It is easy to incorporate bran in a breakfast cereal, for example, but difficulties will arise with lunch and dinner. At that point, you can shift to bran tablets, available in one-gram weights (1000 mgs.), but hypoglycemics are sometimes reluctant to use them because they are made with honey or contain raisins, and because the bran assay shows a considerable amount of carbohydrate. I have not found the amount of honey used to flavor and bind these tablets to be detrimental, and the natural carbohydrate of bran is not utilized by the body. If it were, bran would not be a source of fiber, which by definition is indigestible.

You might start with a teaspoon of bran, added to a whole grain breakfast cereal. At lunch and dinner, take one tablet (1000 mgs.) of bran. Remain at this dosage level for at least a week. This may not solve your constipation problem, but during that period it will at least slow the absorption of the carbohydrates. You may also be troubled by gas during the first week or two. This should not be retained, but should invite a visit to the bathroom. Retained gas exerts almost unbelievable pressure on the colon, and can contribute to the ballooning of segments (diverticulosis).

After a week, gradually increase the amount of bran used, until the criteria for the optimal quantity are met. At that point, the bran intake is not only slowing the absorption of carbohydrate from the intestinal tract, but may be protecting against bowel cancer.

# 10.  The Families of Foods and the Four-Day Rotation Diet

If you are a hypoglycemic, it is very likely that you have food allergies. If you don't, it is certainly important that you do everything possible to avoid them, for they will complicate your troubles with low blood sugar and add new symptoms or intensify old ones.

Allergy to one member of a food family indicates the strong possibility of allergy to other members. Safety to one member may mean safety to others. Knowing which foods are related can help you to avoid unnecessary exposure to foods that may be troublemakers for you. Remember, though, that "may be troublemakers" does not mean that those foods surely will be. You simply should be cautious of them. A person who is strongly allergic to milk, for example, will have to be cautious about cheese, ice cream, and, perhaps, yogurt.

The foods and food families presented in this chapter are listed two ways: first in alphabetical order, which allows you to look up easily any food by name; second, in numerical order, each food family having been assigned a specific number. Beside each food name in the alphabetical list, you will find a number. When you look up that number in the numerical list, you will find that it guides you to the family of foods to which your selection belongs.

The alphabetical and numerical lists of foods can help you to uncover possible allergies, but they also have an opposite purpose. They indicate safer foods. In other words, if you have absolutely no allergic reaction to a member of a food family, chances are good that you will be able to tolerate other foods in that group. Please note my cautious language. I cannot promise you that the failure to react to one food in a family guarantees immunity when you try another one in the same group. Earlier, I cautioned you to remember that allergies can be additive: your allergy to milk, for example, may be so slight that it produces no symptoms, but when you take milk with another food to which you have a slight allergy, the combined effects may be like those of multiplication rather than simple addition.

Intelligent use of the lists provided here should help you markedly in bringing your allergies *to foods* under control. You can also be allergic to anything from plastics to automobile exhaust, from ingredients in paints to synthetic fabrics. These are not within the province of this book, however, and skilled testing and treatment by a qualified bio-ecological allergist are needed. When the symptoms of allergy affect the brain, Vitamin C and Vitamin B6 therapy has been found helpful. For both cerebral allergy and allergy in general, there is a therapy which involves sublingual (under the tongue) administration of free amino acids. The powdered protein acids are held under the tongue for about ten minutes, and then the mixture is swallowed. It tastes remarkably like crab, but its beneficial effects in some highly allergic people make the taste endurable.

One of the by-products of the allergic reaction is a neurotransmitter called "histamine." You are probably aware of this because the use of antihistamine drugs to treat the symptoms of allergy is certainly familiar to the average person. However, these drugs exert their actions only in the blood, and do not reach the histamine stored in the tissues. An elevated level of histamine in the tissues aggravates the problems of allergy and, in addition, may cause depression. Removing excessive amounts of this neurotransmitter from the tissues is a slow process, but it can be accomplished by the regular use of calcium and methionine supplements. The effect of these supplements is to convert histamine into a form that is no longer active in causing the symptoms of allergy. Bioecological allergists are familiar with this action; the orthodox allergist will continue to use the antihistamine drug, however ineffective it may be when the tissue load of histamine is elevated.

# Food Families and Food Family Members (Alphabetical)

## A

| | | | |
|---|---|---|---|
| 81a | abalone | 68 | American persimmon |
| 80 | absinthe | 84 | anchovy |
| 46 | acerola | 84 | Anchovy Family |
| 79 | acorn squash | 65 | angelica |
| 1 | agar | 65 | anise |
| 12 | agave | 38 | annatto |
| 97 | albacore | 133 | antelope |
| 41 | alfalfa | 40a | apple |
| 1 | Algae | 73 | apple mint |
| 63 | allspice | 40b | apricot |
| 40b | almond | 19 | arrowroot (Maranta starch) |
| 11 | *Aloe vera* | 16 | arrowroot (*Musa*) |
| 54 | althaea root | 19 | Arrowroot Family |
| 12 | Amaryllis Family | 80 | artichoke flour |
| 93 | amberjack | 9 | Arum Family |
| 85 | American eel | 11 | asparagus |
| 64 | American ginseng | 34 | avocado |

## B

| | | | |
|---|---|---|---|
| 131 | bacon | 134 | beef |
| 2 | baker's yeast | 134 | beef by-products |
| 6 | bamboo shoots | 134 | beef cattle |
| 16 | banana | 28 | beet |
| 16 | Banana Family | 28 | beet sugar |
| 46 | Barbados cherry | 74 | bell pepper |
| 6 | barley | 73 | bergamot |
| 73 | basil | 11 | Bermuda onion |
| 112 | Bass Family | 23 | Birch Family |
| 53 | basswood | 23 | birch oil |
| 34 | bay leaf | 134 | bison |
| 41 | bean | 38 | Bixa Family |
| 129 | bear | 113 | black bass species |
| 66 | bearberry | 40c | blackberry |
| 129 | Bear Family | 41 | black-eyed pea |
| 24 | Beech Family | 21 | black pepper |
| 24 | beechnut | 40c | black raspberry |

## Food Families and Food Family Members (Alphabetical)

### B

| | | | |
|---|---|---|---|
| 80 | black salsify | 2 | brewer's yeast |
| 22 | black walnut | 41 | broad bean |
| 66 | blueberry | 36 | broccoli |
| 92 | bluefish | 36 | Brussels sprout |
| 92 | Bluefish Family | 27 | buckwheat |
| 113 | bluegill | 27 | Buckwheat Family |
| 80 | boneset | 134 | buffalo |
| 97 | bonito | 109 | buffalofish |
| 71 | borage | 6 | bulgur |
| 71 | Borage Family | 80 | burdock root |
| 79 | Boston marrow | 40d | burnet |
| 134 | Bovine Family | 134 | butter |
| 40c | boysenberry | 31 | Buttercup Family |
| 6 | bran | 79 | buttercup squash |
| 52 | brandy | 100 | butterfish |
| 47 | Brazilian arrowroot | 134 | buttermilk |
| 62 | Brazil nut | 22 | butternut |
| 25 | breadfruit | 79 | butternut squash |

### C

| | | | |
|---|---|---|---|
| 36 | cabbage | 29 | Carpetweed Family |
| 55 | cacao | 1 | carrageen |
| 60 | Cactus Family | 65 | carrot |
| 6 | cane sugar | 65 | Carrot Family |
| 18 | Canna Family | 65 | carrot syrup |
| 79 | cantaloupe | 79 | casaba melon |
| 37 | caper | 48 | cashew |
| 37 | Caper Family | 48 | Cashew Family |
| 42 | carambola | 47 | cassava |
| 65 | caraway seed | 47 | cassava meal |
| 17 | cardamom | 34 | cassia bark and buds |
| 80 | cardoon | 47 | castor bean |
| 132 | caribou | 47 | castor oil |
| 41 | carob | 111 | Catfish Family (freshwater) |
| 41 | carob syrup | 111 | catfish species |
| 110 | carp | 73 | catnip |

| | | | |
|---|---|---|---|
| 36 | cauliflower | 6 | citronella |
| 103 | caviar | 45 | Citrus Family |
| 74 | cayenne pepper | 81c | clam |
| 65 | celeriac | 73 | clary |
| 65 | celery | 63 | clove |
| 65 | celery root | 41 | clover |
| 65 | celery seed and leaf | 81c | cockle |
| 80 | celtuce | 55 | cocoa |
| 9 | ceriman | 55 | cocoa butter |
| 80 | chamomile | 8 | coconut |
| 52 | champagne | 8 | coconut meal |
| 28 | chard | 8 | coconut oil |
| 79 | chayote | 79 | cocozelle |
| 134 | cheese | 86 | cod |
| 32 | cherimoya | 86 | Codfish Family |
| 40b | cherry | 76 | coffee |
| 65 | chervil | 55 | cola nut |
| 24 | chestnut | 36 | collards |
| 67 | chewing gum | 9 | colocasia arrowroot |
| 73 | chia seed | 80 | coltsfoot |
| 122 | chicken | 36 | colza shoots |
| 41 | chick-pea | 71 | comfrey |
| 67 | chicle | 80 | Composite Family |
| 80 | chicory | 5 | Conifer Family |
| 74 | chili pepper | 65 | coriander |
| 36 | Chinese cabbage | 6 | corn |
| 64 | Chinese ginseng | 6 | cornmeal |
| 56 | Chinese gooseberry | 6 | corn oil |
| 14 | Chinese potato | 78 | corn salad |
| 79 | Chinese preserving melon | 6 | cornstarch |
| 7 | Chinese water chestnut | 6 | corn sugar |
| 24 | chinquapin | 6 | corn syrup |
| 11 | chives | 80 | costmary |
| 55 | chocolate | 134 | cottage cheese |
| 110 | chub | 54 | cottonseed oil |
| 7 | chufa | 41 | coumarin |
| 40a | cider | 36 | couve tronchuda |
| 34 | cinnamon | 41 | cowpea |
| 2 | citric acid | 82 | crab |
| 45 | citron | 40a | crabapple |

# Food Families and Food Family Members (Alphabetical)

## C

| | | | |
|---|---|---|---|
| 66 | cranberry | 79 | cucumber |
| 113 | crappie | 65 | cumin |
| 82 | crayfish | 36 | curly tress |
| 52 | cream of tartar | 39 | currant |
| 79 | crenshaw melon | 79 | cushaw squash |
| 95 | croaker | 86 | cusk |
| 115 | Croaker Family (freshwater) | 32 | custard apple |
| 95 | Croaker Family (saltwater) | 32 | Custard-Apple Family |
| 79 | crookneck squash | 4 | Cycad Family |
| 82 | Crustaceans | | |

## D

| | | | |
|---|---|---|---|
| 102 | dab | 73 | dittany |
| 80 | dandelion | 94 | dolphin |
| 9 | dasheen | 94 | Dolphin Family |
| 8 | date | 120 | dove |
| 8 | date sugar | 120 | Dove Family |
| 132 | deer | 52 | dried "currant" |
| 132 | Deer Family | 115 | drum (freshwater) |
| 40c | dewberry | 95 | drum (saltwater) |
| 65 | dill | 119 | Duck Family |
| 56 | Dillenia Family | 119 | duck species |
| 65 | dill seed | 1 | dulse |

## E

| | | | |
|---|---|---|---|
| 17 | East Indian arrowroot | 124 | eggs, turkey |
| 68 | Ebony Family | 77 | elderberry |
| 85 | Eel Family | 77 | elderberry flowers |
| 74 | eggplant | 132 | elk |
| 122 | eggs, chicken | 80 | endive |
| 119 | eggs, duck | 22 | English walnut |
| 119 | eggs, goose | 80 | escarole |
| 123 | eggs, guinea fowl | 63 | eucalyptus |

# Food Families and Food Family Members (Alphabetical)

## H

| | | | |
|---|---|---|---|
| 126 | Hare Family | 6 | hominy grits |
| 100 | harvest fish | 79 | honeydew melon |
| 100 | Harvest Fish Family | 77 | Honeysuckle Family |
| 23 | hazelnut | 25 | hop |
| 22 | heartnut | 73 | horehound |
| 66 | Heath Family | 130 | horse |
| 104 | Herring Family (freshwater) | 130 | Horse Family |
| 83 | Herring Family (saltwater) | 36 | horseradish |
| 54 | hibiscus | 3 | horsetail |
| 22 | hickory nut | 3 | Horsetail Family |
| 90 | hind | 79 | Hubbard squash varieties |
| 131 | hog | 66 | huckleberry |
| 49 | Holly Family | 73 | hyssop |

## I

| | | | |
|---|---|---|---|
| 134 | ice cream | 1 | Irish moss |
| 15 | Iris Family | | |

## J

| | | | |
|---|---|---|---|
| 93 | Jack Family | 80 | Jerusalem artichoke |
| 93 | jack mackerel | 41 | jicama |
| 68 | Japanese persimmon | 5 | juniper |

## K

| | | | |
|---|---|---|---|
| 68 | kaki | 56 | kiwi berry |
| 36 | kale | 36 | kohlrabi |
| 134 | kefir | 36 | kraut |
| 1 | kelp | 41 | kudzu |
| 134 | kid | 45 | kumquat |
| 41 | kidney bean | | |

## L

| | | | |
|---|---|---|---|
| 134 | lactose | | |
| 134 | lamb | 131 | lard |
| 28 | lamb's-quarters | 34 | Laurel Family |

**M**

# Food Families and Food Family Members (Alphabetical)

## N

| | | | |
|---|---|---|---|
| 43 | nasturtium | 96 | northern scup |
| 43 | Nasturtium Family | 33 | nutmeg |
| 41 | navy bean | 33 | Nutmeg Family |
| 40b | nectarine | 2 | nutritional yeast |
| 29 | New Zealand spinach | | |

## O

| | | | |
|---|---|---|---|
| 6 | oat | 125 | opossum |
| 6 | oatmeal | 125 | Opossum Family |
| 87 | ocean catfish | 45 | orange |
| 101 | ocean perch | 20 | Orchid Family |
| 54 | okra | 73 | oregano |
| 134 | oleomargarine | 15 | orrisroot |
| 69 | olive | 42 | oxalis |
| 69 | Olive Family | 42 | Oxalis Family |
| 69 | olive oil | 81c | oyster |
| 11 | onion | 80 | oyster plant |

## P

| | | | |
|---|---|---|---|
| 8 | palm cabbage | 41 | pea |
| 8 | Palm Family | 40b | peach |
| 59 | papain | 122 | peafowl |
| 32 | papaw | 41 | peanut |
| 59 | papaya | 41 | peanut butter |
| 59 | Papaya Family | 41 | peanut oil |
| 74 | paprika | 40a | pear |
| 62 | paradise nut | 22 | pecan |
| 65 | parsley | 40a | pectin |
| 65 | parsnip | 75 | Pedalium Family |
| 121 | partridge | 73 | pennyroyal |
| 58 | Passionflower Family | 74 | pepino |
| 58 | passion fruit | 74 | pepper |
| 6 | patent flour | 21 | peppercorn |
| 79 | pattypan squash | 21 | Pepper Family |

| | | | | |
|---|---|---|---|---|
| 73 | peppermint | | 61 | Pomegranate Family |
| 114 | Perch Family | | 45 | pomelo |
| 79 | Persian melon | | 93 | pompano |
| 122 | pheasant | | 6 | popcorn |
| 122 | Pheasant Family | | 35 | Poppy Family |
| 108 | pickerel | | 35 | poppy seed |
| 120 | pigeon | | 96 | porgy |
| 41 | pigeon pea | | 96 | Porgy Family |
| 30 | pigweed | | 131 | pork |
| 108 | pike | | 131 | pork gelatin |
| 108 | Pike Family | | 74 | potato |
| 83 | pilchard | | 74 | Potato Family |
| 74 | pimiento | | 82 | prawn |
| 10 | pineapple | | 60 | prickly pear |
| 10 | Pineapple Family | | 133 | Pronghorn Family |
| 5 | pine nut | | 26 | Protea Family |
| 5 | piñon | | 40b | prune |
| 41 | pinto bean | | 2 | puffball |
| 48 | pistachio | | 12 | pulque |
| 102 | plaice | | 79 | pumpkin |
| 16 | plantain | | 113 | pumpkinseed (sunfish) |
| 40b | plum | | 79 | pumpkin seed and meal |
| 9 | poi | | 40c | purple raspberry |
| 48 | poison ivy | | 30 | purslane |
| 48 | poison oak | | 30 | Purslane Family |
| 48 | poison sumac | | 16 | psyllium seed |
| 86 | pollack | | 80 | pyrethrum |
| 61 | pomegranate | | | |

**Q**

| | | | | |
|---|---|---|---|---|
| 122 | quail | | 26 | Queensland nut |
| 18 | Queensland arrowroot | | 40a | quince |

**R**

| | | | | |
|---|---|---|---|---|
| 126 | rabbit | | 40c | raspberry |
| 36 | radish | | 40c | raspberry leaf |
| 52 | raisin | | 117 | rattlesnake |
| 11 | ramp | | 6 | raw sugar |
| 36 | rape | | 41 | red clover |

# Food Families and Food Family Members (Alphabetical)

## R

| | | | |
|---|---|---|---|
| 40c | red raspberry | 80 | romaine |
| 90 | red snapper | 40 | Rose Family |
| 132 | reindeer | 101 | rosefish |
| 134 | rennet | 40a | rose hips |
| 134 | rennin | 54 | roselle |
| 27 | rhubarb | 73 | rosemary |
| 6 | rice | 45 | Rue Family |
| 6 | rice flour | 121 | ruffed grouse |
| 90 | rockfish | 36 | rutabaga |
| 134 | Rocky Mountain sheep | 6 | rye |
| 104 | roe | | |

## S

| | | | |
|---|---|---|---|
| 80 | safflower oil | 80 | scolymus |
| 15 | saffron | 101 | Scorpion Fish Family |
| 73 | sage | 80 | scorzonera |
| 8 | sago starch | 131 | scrapple |
| 41 | St.-John's-bread | 86 | scrod |
| 98 | sailfish | 90 | sea bass |
| 105 | Salmon Family | 90 | Sea Bass Family |
| 105 | salmon species | 87 | Sea Catfish Family |
| 80 | salsify | 27 | sea grape |
| 80 | santolina | 83 | sea herring |
| 67 | Sapodilla Family | 95 | sea trout |
| 62 | Sapucaia Family | 1 | seaweed |
| 62 | sapucaia nut | 7 | Sedge Family |
| 83 | sardine | 6 | semolina |
| 11 | sarsaparilla | 41 | senna |
| 34 | sassafras | 75 | sesame butter |
| 114 | sauger | 75 | sesame oil |
| 131 | sausage | 75 | sesame paste |
| 134 | sausage casing | 75 | sesame seed |
| 73 | savory | 104 | shad |
| 39 | Saxifrage Family | 11 | shallot |
| 11 | scallion | 3 | shave grass |
| 81c | scallop | 134 | sheep |

## T

# Food Families and Food Family Members (Alphabetical)

## T

| 47 | tapioca | 41 | tonka bean |
|---|---|---|---|
| 9 | taro | 74 | tree tomato |
| 80 | tarragon | 6 | triticale |
| 57 | tea | 105 | trout species |
| 57 | Tea Family | 2 | truffle |
| 12 | tequila | 97 | tuna |
| 118 | terrapin | 79 | turban squash |
| 73 | thyme | 102 | turbot |
| 91 | tilefish | 124 | turkey |
| 91 | Tilefish Family | 124 | Turkey Family |
| 74 | tobacco | 17 | turmeric |
| 74 | tomatillo | 36 | turnip |
| 74 | tomato | 118 | Turtle Family |
| 86 | tomcod | 118 | turtle species |

## U

| 36 | upland cress |
|---|---|

## V

| 78 | Valerian Family | 132 | venison |
|---|---|---|---|
| 20 | vanilla | 72 | Verbena Family |
| 134 | veal | 41 | vetch |
| 79 | vegetable spaghetti squash | 40a | vinegar |
| 79 | vegetable sponge | | |

## W

| 114 | walleye | 6 | wheat |
|---|---|---|---|
| 22 | Walnut Family | 6 | wheat flour |
| 36 | watercress | 6 | wheat germ |
| 79 | watermelon | 90 | whitebait |
| 41 | wax bean | 106 | whitefish |
| 95 | weakfish | 106 | Whitefish Family |
| 19 | West Indian arrowroot | 21 | white pepper |
| 128 | whale | 112 | white perch |
| 128 | Whale Family | 86 | whiting |

| | | | |
|---|---|---|---|
| 6 | whole wheat flour | 79 | winter melon |
| 6 | wild rice | 73 | winter savory |
| 52 | wine | 80 | witloof chicory |
| 40c | wineberry | 76 | woodruff |
| 52 | wine vinegar | 80 | wormwood |
| 23 | wintergreen | | |

## Y

| | | | |
|---|---|---|---|
| 14 | yam | 114 | yellow perch |
| 14 | Yam Family | 49 | yerba maté |
| 14 | yampi | 134 | yogurt |
| 80 | yarrow | 40c | youngberry |
| 9 | yautia | 47 | yuca |
| 112 | yellow bass | 11 | yucca |
| 93 | yellow jack | | |

## Z

| | |
|---|---|
| 79 | zucchini |

# Food Families (Numerical)

## PLANT

1   Algae
    agar
    carrageen (Irish Moss)
    dulse *
    kelp (seaweed)
2   Fungi
    baker's yeast ("Red Star")
    brewer's yeast (nutritional
  yeast)
    citric acid (*Aspergillus*)
    mold—in certain cheeses
    morel

    mushroom
    puffball
    truffle
3   Horsetail Family, Equi-
  sataceae
    shave grass * (horsetail)
4   Cycad Family, Cycadaceae
    Florida arrowroot (*Zamia*)
5   Conifer Family, Coniferae
    juniper *—used in gin
    pine nut (piñon)

* One or more plant parts (leaf, root, seed, etc.) used as a beverage.

# Food Families (Numerical)

## PLANT

6    Grass Family, Gramineae
       barley
         malt
         maltose
       bamboo shoots
       corn—mature
         cornmeal
         corn oil
         cornstarch
         corn sugar
         corn syrup
         hominy grits
       lemongrass
       millet
       oat
         oatmeal
       popcorn
       rice
         rice flour
       rye
       sorghum grain
         syrup
       sugarcane
         cane sugar
         molasses
         raw sugar
       sweet corn
       triticale
       wheat
         bran (semolina)
         bulgur
         flour
           gluten
           graham
           patent

         whole wheat
         wheat germ
         wild rice
7    Sedge Family, Cyperaceae
       Chinese water chestnut
       chufa (groundnut)
8    Palm Family, Palmaceae
       coconut
         coconut meal
         coconut oil
       date
         date sugar
       palm cabbage
       sago starch (Metroxylon)
9    Arum Family, Araceae
       ceriman (Monstera)
       dasheen (Colocasia ar-
    rowroot)
       malanga (Xanthosoma)
       taro (Colocasia arrowroot)
       poi
       yautia (Xanthosoma)
10   Pineapple Family, Brom-
    eliaceae
       pineapple
11   Lily Family, Liliaceae
       Aloe vera
       asparagus
       chives
       garlic
       leek
       onion
         Bermuda
         Spanish
       ramp

sarsaparilla *
scallion
shallot
yucca (soap plant)
12 Amaryllis Family, Amaryl-
lidaceae
agave
mescal
pulque
tequila
13 Tacca Family, Taccaceae
Fiji arrowroot (*Tacca*)
14 Yam Family, Dioscoreaceae
Chinese potato (yam)
yampi
15 Iris Family, Iridaceae
orrisroot—used in scent
saffron (*Crocus sativus*)
16 Banana Family, Musaceae
arrowroot (*Musa*)
banana
plantain
psyllium seed
17 Ginger Family, Zingiberaceae
cardamom
East Indian arrowroot
(*Curcuma*)
ginger
turmeric
18 Canna Family, Cannaceae
Queensland arrowroot
19 Arrowroot Family, Maran-
taceae
arrowroot (Maranta starch)
20 Orchid Family, Orchidaceae
vanilla

21 Pepper Family, Piperaceae
peppercorn (*Piper*)
22 Walnut Family, Juglandaceae
black walnut
butternut
English walnut
heartnut
hickory nut
pecan
23 Birch Family, Betulaceae
birch oil (wintergreen†)
filbert (hazelnut)
24 Beech Family, Fagaceae
beechnut
chestnut
chinquapin
25 Mulberry Family, Moraceae
breadfruit
fig
hop *
mulberry
26 Protea Family, Proteaceae
macadamia (Queensland
nut)
27 Buckwheat Family, Poly-
gonaceae
buckwheat
garden sorrel
rhubarb
sea grape
28 Goosefoot Family, Che-
nopodiaceae
beet
chard
lamb's-quarters

* One or more plant parts (leaf, root, seed, etc.) used as a beverage.
† Some wintergreen flavor is methyl salicylate.

## Food Families (Numerical)

### PLANT

spinach
sugar beet
beet sugar
tampala
29    Carpetweed Family, Aizoaceae
New Zealand spinach
30    Purslane Family, Portulacaceae
pigweed (purslane)
31    Buttercup Family, Ranunculaceae
goldenseal *
32    Custard-Apple Family, Annonaceae
cherimoya
custard apple
papaw
33    Nutmeg Family, Myristicaceae
mace
nutmeg
34    Laurel Family, Lauraceae
avocado
bay leaf
cassia bark and buds
cinnamon
sassafras *
filé—powdered leaves
35    Poppy Family, Papaveraceae
poppy seed
36    Mustard Family, Cruciferae
broccoli
Brussels sprout
cabbage
kraut
cauliflower
Chinese cabbage
collards
colza shoots
couve tronchuda
curly tress
horseradish
kale
kohlrabi
mustard greens
mustard seed
radish
rape
rutabaga (swede)
turnip
upland cress
watercress
37    Caper Family, Capparidaceae
caper
38    Bixa Family, Bixaceae
annatto—natural yellow dye
39    Saxifrage Family, Saxifragaceae
currant
gooseberry
40    Rose Family, Rosaceae
a. pomes
apple
cider, vinegar
pectin
crabapple
loquat
pear

* One or more plant parts (leaf, root, seed, etc.) used as a beverage.

quince
rose hips *
b. *stone fruits*
almond
apricot
cherry
peach (nectarine)
plum (prune)
sloe
c. *berries*
blackberry
boysenberry
dewberry
loganberry
longberry
raspberry *
black
leaf *
purple
red
strawberry *
leaf *
wineberry
youngberry
d. *herb*
burnet (cucumber flavor)
41   Legume Family, Leguminosae
alfalfa—sprouts *
bean
broad (vetch)
fava
kidney (frijol)
lima
mung—sprouts
navy
pinto
snap
string

wax
black-eyed pea (cowpea)
carob * (locust bean, St.-John's-bread)
carob syrup
chick-pea (garbanzo)
fenugreek *
gum acacia
gum tragacanth
jicama
kudzu
lentil
licorice *
pea
pigeon
snow
peanut (goober)
peanut butter
peanut oil
red clover *
senna *
soybean
lecithin
soy flour
soy grits
soy milk
soy oil
soy sauce (tamari)
tamarind
tonka bean
coumarin
42   Oxalis Family, Oxalidaceae
carambola
oxalis
43   Nasturtium Family, Tropaeolaceae
nasturtium

* One or more plant parts (leaf, root, seed, etc.) used as a beverage.

## Food Families (Numerical)

### PLANT

44    Flax Family, Linaceae
       flaxseed *

45    Rue Family (Citrus Family),
       Rutaceae
       citron
       grapefruit
       kumquat
       lemon
       lime
       mandarin orange
       mandarin tangerine
       murcot
       orange
       pomelo
       tangelo
       tangerine

46    Malpighia Family, Mal-
       pighiaceae
       acerola (Barbados cherry)

47    Spurge Family, Euphor-
       biaceae
       cassava or yuca (*Manihot*)
         cassava meal
         castor bean
         castor oil
         tapioca (Brazilian ar-
rowroot)

48    Cashew Family, Anacar-
       diaceae
       cashew
       mango
       pistachio
       poison ivy
       poison oak
       poison sumac

49    Holly Family, Aquifoliaceae
       maté (yerba maté)

50    Maple Family, Aceraceae
       maple sugar
       maple syrup

51    Soapberry Family, Sapin-
       daceae
       litchi

52    Grape Family, Vitaceae
       grape
         brandy
         champagne
         cream of tartar
         dried "currant"
         raisin
         wine
         wine vinegar
       muscadine

53    Linden Family, Tiliaceae
       basswood * (linden)

54    Mallow Family, Malvaceae
       althaea root *
       cottonseed oil
       hibiscus * (roselle)
       okra

55    Sterculia Family, Ster-
       culiaceae
       chocolate * (cacao)
       cocoa *
         cocoa butter
       cola nut

56    Dillenia Family, Dilleniaceae
       Chinese gooseberry (kiwi
berry)

57    Tea Family, Theaceae
       tea *

* One or more plant parts (leaf, root, seed, etc.) used as a beverage.

58 Passionflower Family, Passifloraceae
   granadilla (passion fruit)
59 Papaya Family, Caricaceae
   papain
   papaya
60 Cactus Family, Cactaceae
   prickly pear
61 Pomegranate Family, Punicaceae
   pomegranate
   grenadine
62 Sapucaia Family, Lecythidaceae
   Brazil nut
   sapucaia nut (paradise nut)
63 Myrtle Family, Myrtaceae
   allspice (*Pimenta*)
   clove
   eucalyptus *
   guava
64 Ginseng Family, Araliaceae
   American ginseng *
   Chinese ginseng *
65 Carrot Family, Umbelliferae
   angelica
   anise
   caraway seed
   carrot
     carrot syrup
   celeriac (celery root)
   celery
     celery seed and leaf *
   chervil
   coriander
   cumin
   dill
     dill seed
   fennel *

   finocchio (Florence fennel)
   gotu kola *
   lovage *
   parsley *
   parsnip
   sweet cicely
66 Heath Family, Ericaceae
   bearberry *
   blueberry *
   cranberry
   huckleberry *
67 Sapodilla Family, Sapotaceae
   chicle (chewing gum)
68 Ebony Family, Ebonaceae
   American persimmon
   kaki (Japanese persimmon)
69 Olive Family, Oleaceae
   olive—green or ripe
   olive oil
70 Morning Glory Family, Convolvulaceae
   sweet potato
71 Borage Family, Boraginaceae (Herbs)
   borage
   comfrey—leaf and root *
72 Verbena Family, Verbenaceae
   lemon verbena *
73 Mint Family, Labiatae (Herbs)
   apple mint
   basil
   bergamot
   catnip *
   chia seed *
   clary
   dittany *
   horehound *

* One or more plant parts (leaf, root, seed, etc.) used as a beverage.

## Food Families (Numerical)

### PLANT

hyssop *
lavender
lemon balm *
marjoram
oregano
pennyroyal *
peppermint *
rosemary
sage
spearmint *
summer savory
thyme
winter savory

74 Potato Family, Solanaceae
eggplant
ground-cherry
pepino (melon pear)
pepper (*Capsicum*)
bell (sweet)
cayenne
chili
paprika
pimiento
potato
tobacco
tomatillo
tomato
tree tomato

75 Pedalium Family, Pedaliaceae
sesame seed
sesame butter
sesame oil
sesame paste

76 Madder Family, Rubiaceae
coffee *

woodruff

77 Honeysuckle Family, Caprifoliaceae
elderberry
elderberry flowers *

78 Valerian Family, Valerianaceae
corn salad (fetticus)

79 Gourd Family, Cucurbitaceae
chayote
Chinese preserving melon
cucumber
gherkin
loofah (vegetable sponge)
muskmelon
cantaloupe
casaba
crenshaw
honeydew
Persian
winter
pumpkin
pumpkin seed and meal
squash
acorn
buttercup
butternut
Boston marrow
cocozelle
crookneck
straightneck
cushaw
golden nugget
Hubbard varieties
pattypan

* One or more plant parts (leaf, root, seed, etc.) used as a beverage.

turban
vegetable spaghetti
zucchini
watermelon
80 Composite Family, Compositae
boneset *
burdock root *
cardoon
chamomile
chicory *
coltsfoot
costmary
dandelion
endive
escarole
globe artichoke
goldenrod *
Jerusalem artichoke
artichoke flour

lettuce
celtuce
pyrethrum
romaine
safflower oil
salsify (oyster plant)
santolina (herb)
scolymus (Spanish oyster plant)
scorzonera (black salsify)
southernwood
sunflower
sunflower seed, meal, and oil
tansy (herb)
tarragon (herb)
witloof chicory (French endive)
wormwood (absinthe)
yarrow *

## ANIMAL

81 Mollusks
  *a. gastropods*
    abalone
    snail
  *b. cephalopod*
    squid
  *c. pelecypods*
    clam
    cockle
    mussel
    oyster
    scallop
82 Crustaceans
    crab
    crayfish
    lobster

prawn
shrimp

*Saltwater Fishes*

83 Herring Family
    menhaden
    pilchard (sardine)
    sea herring
84 Anchovy Family
    anchovy
85 Eel Family
    American eel
86 Codfish Family
    cod (scrod)
    cusk

* One or more plant parts (leaf, root, seed, etc.) used as a beverage.

## ANIMAL

      haddock
      hake
      pollack
      silver hake
      tomcod
      whiting

87    Sea Catfish Family
      ocean catfish

88    Mullet Family
      mullet

89    Silversides Family
      silversides (whitebait)

90    Sea Bass Family
      grouper
      hind
      red snapper
      rockfish
      sea bass
      spotted bass
      striped bass

91    Tilefish Family
      tilefish

92    Bluefish Family
      bluefish

93    Jack Family
      amberjack
      jack mackerel
      pompano
      yellow jack

94    Dolphin Family
      dolphin

95    Croaker Family
      croaker
      drum
      sea trout
      silver perch
      spot
      weakfish (spotted sea trout)

96    Porgy Family
      northern scup (porgy)

97    Mackerel Family
      albacore
      bonito
      mackerel
      skipjack
      tuna

98    Marlin Family
      marlin
      sailfish

99    Swordfish Family
      swordfish

100   Harvest Fish Family
      butterfish
      harvest fish

101   Scorpion Fish Family
      rosefish (ocean perch)

102   Flounder Family
      dab
      flounder
      halibut
      plaice
      sole
      turbot

*Freshwater Fishes*

103   Sturgeon Family
      sturgeon
      caviar

104   Herring Family
      shad
      roe

105   Salmon Family
      salmon species
      trout species

106   Whitefish Family
      whitefish

107    Smelt Family
     smelt
108    Pike Family
     muskellunge
     pickerel
     pike
109    Sucker Family
     buffalofish
     sucker
110    Minnow Family
     carp
     chub
111    Catfish Family
     catfish species
112    Bass Family
     white perch
     yellow bass
113    Sunfish Family
     black bass species
     bluegill
     crappie
     sunfish species
     pumpkinseed
114    Perch Family
     sauger
     walleye
     yellow perch
115    Croaker Family
     drum

*Amphibians*

116    Frog Family
     frog
      frogs' legs

*Reptiles*

117    Snake Family
     rattlesnake

118    Turtle Family
     terrapin
     turtle species

*Birds*

119    Duck Family
     duck species
      eggs
     goose
     greylag
      eggs
120    Dove Family
     dove
     pigeon (squab)
121    Grouse Family
     ruffed grouse (partridge)
122    Pheasant Family
     chicken
      eggs
     peafowl
     pheasant
     quail
123    Guinea Fowl Family
     guinea fowl
      eggs
124    Turkey Family
     turkey
      eggs

*Mammals*

125    Opossum Family
     opossum
126    Hare Family
     rabbit
127    Squirrel Family
     squirrel

**ANIMAL**

128    Whale Family
    whale
129    Bear Family
    bear
130    Horse Family
    horse
131    Swine Family
    hog (pork)
    bacon
    ham
    lard
    pork gelatin
    sausage
    scrapple
132    Deer Family
    caribou
    deer (venison)
    elk
    moose
    reindeer
133    Pronghorn Family
    antelope
134    Bovine Family
    beef cattle
    beef

beef by-products
    gelatin
    margarine
    rennin (rennet)
    sausage casing
    suet
milk products
    butter
    buttermilk
    cheese
    cottage cheese
    ice cream
    kefir
    lactose
    spray dried milk
    yogurt
    veal
buffalo (bison)
goat (kid)
    cheese
    ice cream
    milk
Rocky Mountain sheep
sheep—domestic
    lamb
    mutton

## The Four-Day Rotation Diet

On a rotation diet you use foods to which you are not allergic or to which your allergic reactions are very mild, and you also refrain from repeating foods often enough to become allergic to them. The four-day interval before repeating a food seems to be the minimum that will confer such protection.

A strong addiction to a food, whether or not you are conscious of it, is frequently a token of allergic addiction. Since the foods to which you are addicted are most likely those you eat most frequently, this is an important phenomenon. The situation is parallel to that of a drug addict, who takes the drug not only because he wants a high, but because he desperately wants to avoid a low (withdrawal symptoms). There are also withdrawal symptoms when you stop eating a food to which you are allergically addicted, and, conversely, there are temporary dividends when you do eat that food. Many allergic individuals are unconscious of this mechanism. The technician in nutrition, if challenged to test for allergy in a minimum period of time, will simply ask the patient what foods he likes the most and eats the most frequently. He will then tell the patient to stop eating them. The law of averages will have him on target more frequently than you would suppose. This is the rationale for a rotation diet.

As you read the sample menus I provide and the lists of food families from which the menus are drawn, you will become conscious of a problem which is very difficult to solve. Simply, this: when a person with low blood sugar also has multiple allergies (not an infrequent combination of troubles), the nutritional and menu requirements for the two disorders frequently collide. For example, citrus fruit is one of the food families from which I draw on the first day (assuming, of course, no allergy to citrus). However, oranges and grapefruit contain 10 percent sugar, which may be an overdose for a hypoglycemic. Those with mild allergies and mild hypoglycemia are able to manage this problem. When the symptoms of both disorders are severe, however, choices from the food families obviously must be more restricted. Not infrequently, patients have come to me, weeping, because they didn't know what they could eat. But don't assume that the nutritionist will always be able to solve the problem completely. Allergists who recognize the existence and the effects of food allergy do not all have the same system for scoring the presence, the severity, or the absence of allergy. If you are faced with the job of assembling menus in which foods will be rotated, it is essential that you know the battle plan of your allergist. There will be foods he will want you to avoid for at least a year; some he will want you to taboo for at least six months; some he is willing to have you repeat every seven days; and some with which he will want a four-day rotation. One instruction, though, is almost universal: don't fall in love with a food, even if you are completely free of any allergic reaction to it. Repetition here does not add emphasis—it creates an allergy.

This warning clearly applies to the sweet tooth, for indulging that is the first step toward low blood sugar and the tendency to allergy. Sugar is one of the five causes of hypoglycemia, which I call "SCAMS," for sugar, caffeine, allergy, malnourishment, and stress. And the craving for sugar is an excellent example of allergic addiction. One effect of sugar, among many others, is a rise in the brain level of a neurotransmitter, serotonin. This is a quieting neurotransmitter for most hypoglycemics. The person with the sweet tooth is not aware that his "sugar fix" gives him some transient peace and quiet, as a result of the rise in his calmative neurotransmitter serotonin. He is likely to be aware, though, that when deprived of his favorite sweetener, he is nervous. The knowledgeable nutritionist will take advantage of this mechanism by triggering it with a protein—the amino acid tryptophan. Tryptophan is used by the body as a precursor of two factors: serotonin and niacinamide. To discourage niacinamide production, the vitamin is given with tryptophan. A moderate amount of Vitamin B6 is also needed and administered in this biochemical reaction. The net result is the same rise in serotonin levels formerly provided by sugar, but created by a protein, which for the hypoglycemic is a much better pathway.

You may wonder if the food families and the four-day rotation diet are worth the effort. Certainly, not all hypoglycemics are allergic, and not all of those with allergies need this Draconian discipline. But for some of those who do need it, these nutritional devices have been the only way back to health.

## Four-Day Rotation Diet

*Food Families: Day 1*

*Pineapple*   Pineapple
*Palm*   Coconut, date, date sugar
*Citrus*   Lemon, orange, grapefruit, lime, tangerine, kumquat, citron, tangelo, mandarin orange, mandarin tangerine
*Buckwheat*   Buckwheat, rhubarb
*Mustard*   Mustard, mustard greens, turnip, kohlrabi, Brussels sprouts, radish, horseradish, watercress, cabbage (red or white), kraut, cauliflower, kale, collards, broccoli

*Birch*   Filbert, hazelnut
*Morning Glory*   Sweet potato
*Yam*   Yam
*Olive*   Black or green olives
*Potato*   Pimiento
*Myrtle*   Allspice, cloves, guava
*Ginseng*   Ginseng root
*Bovine*   Beef, veal, lamb, goat; dairy products (butter, cheese, cottage cheese, yogurt, kefir, buttermilk, milk)
*Salmon*   Salmon, trout
*Turkey*
*Tea*   Comfrey, ginseng
*Oil*   Butter, olive oil
*Sweetener*   Date sugar, fructose
*Juice*   Juices (unsweetened) may be made from any of the fruits or vegetables listed above. Juices are rich in sugar, and it may be necessary to limit sharply the intake of citrus, as whole fruit or as juice. This is, of course, a consideration for hypoglycemics, though such fruits in reasonable quantities may present no problems for those who are not allergic to them.

*Sample Diet: Day 1*

BREAKFAST

4 ounces orange juice\* or 1 cup fresh pineapple slices, orange slices
Bowl (⅓ cup dry) of buckwheat (kasha) cereal with 1 pat butter†
and 1 teaspoon date sugar
Ginseng tea

MIDMORNING SNACK

2 ounces filberts
4 or 5 dates

---

\* Juice should be unsweetened (preferably fresh-squeezed). Remember that high intake of juices, even when unsweetened, can touch off hypoglycemic symptoms in persons with severe low blood sugar.

LUNCH

3 ounces lean veal* or fowl (turkey without skin)
½ cup steamed cauliflower with 1 ounce melted cheddar
½ cup baked sweet potato or yam with 1 pat butter†
1 cup steamed greens (mustard, turnip, kale, or collards)
6 to 8 green olives stuffed with pimientos
6 raw radishes
1 cup yogurt with 2 ounces shredded coconut

MIDAFTERNOON SNACK

Tangerine or tangelo

DINNER

4 ounces broiled salmon or trout or 4 ounces lean beef or lamb*
1 cup steamed Brussels sprouts or broccoli with 1 pat butter†
1 cup steamed cabbage or kohlrabi
*Salad:*
    ½ cup shredded red cabbage
    ½ cup watercress
    6 black olives
    2 ounces cottage cheese†

*Dressing:*
    1 tablespoon olive oil and ¼ lemon (juice)
    ½ cup mandarin oranges or guava
    1 glass (6 ounces) milk or buttermilk

NIGHT SNACK

2 ounces hazelnuts

---

* Horseradish or mustard may be used as a sauce for meat.
† If possible, dairy products should be made from raw certified milk (sometimes available at health-food stores).

*Food Families: Day 2*

*Banana*   Banana, plantain, psyllium seed
*Honeysuckle*   Elderberry
*Saxifrage*   Currants, gooseberry
*Heath*   Blueberry, huckleberry, bearberry, cranberry
*Birch*   Wintergreen
*Grape*   Grapes (all varieties), raisins
*Holly*   Maté
*Walnut*   English walnut, black walnut, pecan, hickory nut, butternut
*Goosefoot*   Beet, spinach, chard, lamb's-quarters (greens), sugar beet
*Pedalium*   Sesame seed, sesame paste, sesame oil, sesame butter
*Carrot*   Carrot, parsnip, parsley, celery, celery seed, celeriac, anise,
   dill, fennel, cumin, coriander, caraway, chervil
*Fungi*   Mushroom
*Beech*   Beechnut, chestnut
*Pheasant*   Chicken, quail, peafowl, pheasant, chicken eggs
*Flounder*   Flounder, halibut
*Codfish*   Cod, haddock, pollack, tomcod, silver hake
*Crustaceans*   Prawn, crayfish
*Mollusks*   Clams, mussels, oysters, scallops, cockles
*Tea*   Elderberry, blueberry, bearberry, fennel
*Oil*
*Sweetener*   Beet sugar, honey
*Juice*   Juices (unsweetened) can be made from any of the fruits or
   vegetables listed above. Remember that high intake of juices, even
   when unsweetened, can touch off hypoglycemia symptoms in persons
   with severe low blood sugar.

*Sample Diet: Day 2*
                    BREAKFAST
4 ounces unsweetened grape juice
Raisin and nut cereal *
1 sliced banana
Blueberry tea

---

* Raisin and nut cereal: 2 ounces raisins and 3 ounces nuts (walnuts, pecans, hickory nuts, butternuts, beechnuts, psyllium seeds), ground to make fine cereal.

MIDMORNING SNACK

Handful (1 ounce) hickory nuts
1 cup fresh blueberries


LUNCH

4 ounces broiled fish (codfish family), shellfish, * or mushroom
    omelette (2 eggs without milk)
1 cup baked parsnips or plantains
1 cup steamed beets
*Salad:*
        1 cup raw spinach
        ½ cup raw chervil
        ½ cup sliced mushrooms

*Dressing:*
        1 tablespoon sesame oil and fresh dill
        ½ cup chestnut puree (sweetened with honey)

Fennel tea


MIDAFTERNOON SNACK

Handful (1 ounce) of pecans
2 ounces of currants†


DINNER

1 glass (8 ounces) fresh carrot juice with 1–2 ounces parsley or
    spinach juice
4 ounces lean fowl (pheasant family) without skin or fish
    (flounder, halibut) with ¼ cup cranberry sauce (sweetened
    with honey)
1 cup steamed chard or lamb's-quarters
1 cup steamed carrots with parsley


* Prawn, crayfish, clams, mussels, oysters, scallops, cockles.
† Dried fruits may be unsulphured (available at health-food stores).

*Salad:*
> celery and carrot sticks
> raw fennel
> 2 teaspoons tahini (sesame paste) or sesame butter and
> herbs

1 cup grapes

NIGHT SNACK

Elderberry tea

*Food Families: Day 3*

*Rose*   Strawberry, raspberry, blackberry, loganberry, youngberry, boy-senberry, rose hip, apple, pear, quince, plum, prune, cherry, peach, apricot, nectarine, almond, wild cherry

*Ebony*   Persimmon

*Protea*   Macadamia nut

*Conifer*   Pine nut

*Flax*   Flaxseed

*Legume*   Black-eyed pea, carob (St. John's bread, locust bean) fava bean, broad bean (vetch), alfalfa, garbanzo (chick-pea), snap bean, goober, green pea, kidney bean (frijol), lentil, licorice, lima bean, mung bean, navy bean, peanut (butter and oil), pigeon pea, pinto bean, soybean, soy flour, lecithin, soy oil, string bean, tamarind, wax bean, snow pea, sprouts (mung, soybean, lentil, chick-pea, alfalfa), tamari (soy sauce)

*Grass*   Wheat, corn, rice, oats, oatmeal, barley, malt, rye, wild rice, millet, sorghum, molasses, bamboo shoots, sugarcane, sprouts (wheat)

*Lily*   Onion, garlic, asparagus, chive, leek, Bermuda onion, shallot, scallion, Spanish onion

*Sedge*   Chinese water chestnut

*Arrowroot*   Maranta starch

*Ginger*   Ginger, turmeric

*Iris*   Saffron (flower and seed)

*Duck*   Mallard duck, greylag goose

*Swine*   Pork, pork products
*Crustaceans*   Crab, lobster, shrimp
*Mollusks*   Abalone, snails, squid, clams, mussels
*Flounder*   Sole
*Bass*   Striped bass, rockfish, spotted bass, grouper, hind, white perch
*Sunfish*   Largemouth and smallmouth black bass, spotted black bass, black sea bass, sunfish, pumpkinseed, bluegill

*Tea*   Rose hip, alfalfa, licorice root
*Oil*   Soybean, peanut, flaxseed
*Sweetener*   Carob syrup, tupelo or wildflower honey (if honey was not used on another day of rotation), molasses, sorghum
*Juice*   Juices (unsweetened) may be made from any of the fruits and vegetables listed above, including sprouts. Remember that high intake of juices, even when unsweetened, can touch off hypoglycemic symptoms in persons with severe low blood sugar.

*Sample Diet: Day 3*

### BREAKFAST

Bowl (⅓ cup dry) of millet or oatmeal with 1 teaspoon molasses and 1 teaspoon ground flaxseed
⅓ cup prunes or dried apricots *
Rose hip or alfalfa tea

### MIDMORNING SNACK

1 ounce macadamia nuts or pine nuts
1 apple

### LUNCH

4 ounces steamed shrimp, crab meat, or broiled fish (flounder, bass, or sunfish family)
2 cups Chinese vegetables sautéed with ½ cup tofu (bamboo shoots, water chestnuts, scallions, onions, snowpeas, mung sprouts, soybean sprouts, fresh ginger), and with 1 tablespoon arrowroot starch for thickening

---

* Dried fruits should be unsulphured.

½ cup brown rice or wild rice
1 persimmon or pear
Rose hip tea

MIDAFTERNOON SNACK
2 rice cakes with 2 teaspoons fresh peanut butter* or handful (1 ounce) raw almonds

DINNER
1 cup pea or lentil soup
4 ounces lean pork, broiled shellfish (lobster, abalone, squid, snails), or broiled fish (sole, bass, or black bass family), or 4 ounces broiled fowl (mallard duck, greylag goose) without skin, or 6 ounces steamed squid, clams, or mussels
Fresh corn on the cob (1 ear) or ½ cup pearl barley
1 cup steamed asparagus
*Sprout salad:*
    2 cups fresh sprouts (alfalfa, lentil, wheat, chick-pea, or mung)
    ¼ cup chopped chives or shallots

*Dressing:*
    1 tablespoon soybean or peanut oil, fresh ginger, minced, and tamari (soy sauce)†

1 cup fresh strawberries

NIGHT SNACK
Licorice tea

*Food Families: Day 4*

*Mulberry*    Mulberry, fig, breadfruit
*Custard-Apple*    Papaw, cherimoya

---

* Buy peanut butter freshly ground at your health-food store to avoid additives.
† Tamari (soy sauce) may be used for flavoring.

*Papaya*   Papaya, papain
*Gourd*   Watermelon, cantaloupe, winter melon and other melons, pumpkin, cucumber, squash, pumpkin and squash seeds
*Cashew*   Cashew, pistachio, mango
*Sapucaia*   Brazil nut
*Mallow*   Okra, cottonseed
*Potato*   Potato, tomato, eggplant, sweet and bell pepper, paprika, cayenne
*Pepper*   Black and white pepper, peppercorns
*Composite*   Lettuce, chicory, endive, escarole, globe artichoke, Jerusalem artichoke, dandelion, sunflower seeds and oil, tarragon, safflower oil, chamomile, goldenrod
*Laurel*   Avocado, cinnamon, bay leaf, sassafras, cassia buds or cassia bark
*Nutmeg*   Nutmeg, mace
*Spurge*   Tapioca
*Orchid*   Vanilla
*Maple*   Maple sugar and syrup
*Mint*   Basil, summer savory, sage, oregano, horehound, catnip, spearmint, peppermint, thyme, marjoram, lemon balm
*Grouse*
*Guinea Fowl*
*Dove*   Pigeon
*Herring*   Herring, shad, sardine
*Whitefish*
*Mackerel*   Mackerel, tuna, bonito
*Porgy*
*Codfish*   Whiting
*Bluefish*
*Jack*   Pompano, amberjack, jack mackerel
*Sea Bass*   Red snapper
*Croaker*   Weakfish, croaker, freshwater drum
*Sturgeon*
*Anchovy*
*Harvest Fish*   Butterfish
*Tea*   Mint, sassafras, papaya, chamomile, fennel, peppermint
*Oil*   Cottonseed, sunflower seed, safflower oil

*Sweetener*   Maple sugar and syrup, avocado honey, sage honey (if honey was not used on another day of rotation)

*Juice*   Juices (unsweetened) may be made from any of the fruits or vegetables listed above, including tea herbs and melons. Remember that high intake of juices, even when unsweetened, can touch off hypoglycemic symptoms in persons with severe low blood sugar.

## Sample Diet: Day 4

### BREAKFAST
4 ounces unsweetened papaya juice
1 cup fresh mango and papaya slices
Fig and nut cereal* with 1 teaspoon maple syrup
Papaya or chamomile tea

### MIDMORNING SNACK
2 ounces pistachio nuts or sunflower seeds
1 cup cherimoyas or ½ fresh papaya

### LUNCH
8 ounces fresh tomato juice or tomato-cucumber juice
3 ounces tuna, herring, or sardines
½ cup baked squash (butternut or acorn)
*Salad:*
      1 cup romaine or Boston lettuce
      ½ cucumber, sliced
      ½ zucchini, sliced
      3 or 4 Jerusalem artichokes, sliced
      ½ ripe avocado

*Dressing:*
      1 tablespoon safflower oil and herbs (basil, thyme, tarragon, or marjoram)

Sassafras tea

* Fig and nut cereal: 2 ounces chopped figs and 2 ounces nuts and seeds (cashews, Brazil nuts; sunflower seeds, pumpkin and squash seeds), ground to a fine cereal.

MIDAFTERNOON SNACK

½ cantaloupe, small honeydew, casaba, or other melon, or 4 inch × 4 inch wedge of watermelon

DINNER

6 ounces fresh tomato juice
4 ounces broiled or baked fish* or 4 ounces broiled fowl (grouse, guinea fowl, or pigeon) without skin
1 medium baked potato
1 cup stewed okra and eggplant with tomatoes
*Salad:*
    6 artichoke hearts
    1 cup escarole and endive
    ½ cup dandelion leaves
    Sweet and bell pepper slices

*Dressing:*
    1 tablespoon sunflower seed oil, ½ avocado (mashed), herbs
    ½ cup tapioca (vanilla, sweetened with maple sugar)

NIGHT SNACK

Fennel or peppermint tea

---

*Whitefish, mackerel family, porgy, bluefish, jack, red snapper, whiting, croaker family, sturgeon, harvest fish.

# 11.   Mercury Aggravates the Symptoms of Hypoglycemia

The dark metallic filling in your teeth is 40 to 50 percent mercury, which is alien to the body. One dentist has shown that for a period of up to one hundred days after a filling is installed, the body reacts by producing, in adjacent tissue, "foreign body giant cell reactions," which demonstrate that mercury amalgam is alien and certainly not wholly acceptable to the body. As you chew, mercury vapor may be released from the fillings and absorbed by your body. Both of these statements are based on actual tests: there is an instrument that measures the amount of mercury vapor released after hard chewing, and there are tests for the absorption of mercury by the body. To complicate matters, the mouth bacteria that are blamed for plaque are capable of converting ordinary mercury into methyl mercury. Methyl mercury is so toxic that it caused alarm in scientific circles a few years ago when it was found to be the form of the poison carried in some varieties of fish. Mercury is not only toxic, but it has an affinity for proteins. It therefore attaches itself to blood cells, interferes with the function of the glands, and acts as a poison for the nervous system and the brain. In addition, it has potentially vicious effects on the lungs, the heart, the liver, and the kidneys. There is also one indirect effect, which may be the most threatening of all: mercury depresses the immune system. Since that system is responsible for resistance to infection and to cancer, that action of mercury should prompt readers who have such fillings into seeking examination for mercury retention and toxicity.

Hair analysis has been enthusiastically recommended for determination of nutritional and toxic metal analysis. Interpretation of the results is difficult, however. Does a high level of mercury in the hair reflect a high level in the body, or does it represent successful excretion, the body thereby ridding itself of the poison? The other side of the coin raises the same question: does a low hair level accurately reflect a low level in the body, or does it mean that the tissues are clinging to this burden of mercury which refuses to leave?

In the alternative therapies clinic with which I am associated, our first of possibly four tests is for release of mercury vapor after chewing. The second test is an electrical one. When you mix different metals, and place them in an electrolyte solution (saliva), electrogalvanic currents may be released. If current is present, then whether it is positive or negative will determine the sequence in which the mercury amalgam will be removed. Removal in improper sequence can cause severe symptoms in sensitive patients. We are compelled to conjecture on the effect of such electro-activity in the mouth, at the base of the brain. Acupuncturists say, for example, that it may cause or aggravate the symptoms of temporomandibular joint dysfunction (TMJ), among other mischief. The next test is analysis of a twenty-four-hour urine sample for mercury. Here again, a low level may mean tissue retention rather than freedom from mercury in the body. But the fourth test, also performed on the urine, finally gives the definitive answer. It follows a month of treatment with nutrients that displace mercury in the body, using some that are largely sulfur compounds, since sulfur is an antagonist of mercury. We employ selenium, L-cysteine, and glutathione, which we found to be effective, although some clinics and medical groups use doses of metals as antagonists to mercury. If at the end of a month of antimercury treatment the excretion of mercury rises sharply, the diagnosis is established. The cysteine-selenium-glutathione treatment is not necessarily stopped when the mercury excretion reaches an irreducible low. All three nutrients are antioxidants, and antioxidants generally are anti-aging and anticancer.

Let's follow a typical patient through this procedure. She has come to the medical-nutritional center because she is suffering from multiple allergies and has a tendency toward weight gain out of proportion to the amount of food she is eating. Carbohydrates are her particular enemy, for on a binge of starch and sugar she can gain as much as six to eight pounds in three days. She complains of depression, which ordinarily might be easily assignable to her troubles, but proves at least in part to be physical in origin. She also has a history of repeated vaginal yeast infections. The final insult is a series of panic attacks, with tremendous anxiety coming out of the blue and nothing in her life situation to justify it. These attacks leave her drenched with perspiration and unable to function.

A glucose-tolerance test is ordered, but I am wary of her response to a dose of sugar and ask the nurse to remain in the room for the full six hours. The patient's glucose tolerance is normal to the fourth hour, but then she develops a violent panic attack, has a mild convulsion, and would have fallen off the table if the nurse had not been there.

Repeated yeast infections are common in patient histories. Superficially, what triggers migration of yeast to the vagina is a medication, such as antibiotics, cortisone, the birth control pill, or some similar insult. Sometimes stress does it—the initiation of the menses, childbirth, or a period of violent emotional tension. Sometimes mercury toxicity does it. We are all infected with yeast, but only in a minority does the organism begin vigorously to colonize the tissues. When it reaches the gut, it can damage the wall, which may permit the absorption of foods before they are completely digested. *There* is the start of the multiple allergies. As you know from the use of antihistamines for allergy symptoms, there are drugs that reduce blood levels of histamine. Unfortunately, they don't have the same effect on histamine in the tissues. When this neurotransmitter collects in the tissues, it can cause suicidal depression.

A complaint of the patient that would have been taken seriously by any practitioner familiar with mercury poisoning was a constant feeling of being cold. This had been reported to her previous physicians, who dropped the hunt for the cause after determining that the thyroid gland was functioning normally. In fact, the interference of mercury with the thyroid hormone is not at the level of the gland itself but at the cellular level. When the mercury has been dispossessed, the temperature usually returns to normal, sometimes in a matter of days.

The patient was told to begin the expensive and uncomfortable process of having the amalgam removed from her teeth. Simultaneously, she was placed on a low-carbohydrate, high-protein, high-fat diet. This choice was dictated by three considerations: her easy weight gain from carbohydrates, her low blood sugar, and the need to discourage yeast (which thrives on sugar). The diet was supplemented with the antimercury nutrients and with those used to dispossess yeast, including lactobacillus bacteria, garlic, and biotin. Nutrients were also employed to stimulate the immune system, since that is depressed by mercury. The patient also took a tablespoon of edible-grade linseed oil daily, which supplies a type of fatty acid that encourages weight loss on a low-carbohydrate diet. A Vitamin B Complex supplement was prescribed to help liver function, usually critical to the recovery from hypoglycemia.

After six weeks on this regimen, the patient reported that she had lost fifteen pounds between a Friday night and a Monday morning. Her depression markedly lessened. Supplements of calcium and methionine slowly brought down the remaining tissue histamine, and when that reached a low level, the rest of her depression vanished. The multiple allergies weakened, and the yeast infection gradually yielded—in its final stages, it became necessary to use an antiyeast drug.

This history gives you a picture of the remote consequences of what would appear to be minor errors in diet. Consider that hypoglycemia is frequently triggered by excessive consumption of sugar and refined starches. Such a diet is conducive to tooth decay, which brings the amalgam into the scene. The mercury toxicity from the amalgam ultimately triggers the yeast infection, and that in turn starts the allergies.

Both syphilis and low blood sugar have been called the "great imitators" because their symptoms may suggest those of many other disorders. Mercury poisoning should be added to the list. I have seen patients who were not hypoglycemic but had all the symptoms, because of chronic mercury toxicity. Narcolepsy was the diagnosis that proved erroneous in a man who fell asleep in the middle of conversations. His problem was mercury toxicity. A forty-four-year-old man with severe muscle weakness, to the point where he had to wear braces on his legs, was originally diagnosed as suffering from multiple sclerosis. There was no improvement when his mercury analgam was removed, but his steady downward course was halted. The case closely paralleled ones with a more dramatic response, reported by Dr. Hal Huggins, DDS, in a monograph on mercury poisoning.

Needless to say, children are also subject to mercury poisoning from amalgam. Some children carry a burden not only of mercury, but of arsenic, cadmium, and aluminum, and it is very difficult, if not impossible at times, to track down the sources of these poisons. But it is rewarding when a child can be taken off stimulant drugs as his "hyperactivity" improves on appropriate nutritional therapy and, where needed, the removal of mercury from his small body.

As the American Medical Association has tried to discourage the profession and the public from investigating hypoglycemia, the American Dental Association (ADA) has reacted to amalgam research by denying that amalgam releases mercury. The society should look at its own history, for it sprang from the ashes of the original dental society, which was destroyed by an intramural fight about the dangers of amalgam. American Dental Association speakers tried recently to minimize the problem of amalgam by calling it "sensationalism in the media." They then announced that mercury *is* released, but that the problem is self-limited, because ultimately the mercury is all vaporized. That, of course, leaves the question—where did it go? In any event, said an ADA spokesman, only those hypersensitive to mercury would be in any danger, and those patients, to quote him, "are a very small minority." No one asked the logical question: "How do you know they are a very small minority?" Mercury sensitivity testing is certainly not a practice in the vast majority of dental offices.

One troubled dentist wrote to the society with a scathing question. "You tell practitioners that we must protect ourselves, when we work with amalgam, from inhaling the vapor. We are told to be careful in storing it, lest elevated room temperature release mercury vapors. From all this, am I to gather that the only safe place to store the amalgam is in our patients' mouths?" The dental society ducked the issue by declaring that the two situations are not parallel. It is reminiscent of the tactic used by the American Medical Association, which found hypoglycemia symptoms so frequent, despite its protestations of their rarity, that it finally labeled the phenomenon "idiopathic postprandial syndrome." This means symptoms, after eating, of unknown origin. Unknown only to the AMA.

Some dentists are troubled by the choice of materials to use in place of amalgam. Gold is a frequent first choice, but obviously is expensive. There are "composites" available, which are perfectly satisfactory. Scotch P-30 is reported to be excellent. A frequent question from the layman is "Couldn't I keep my amalgam, and use the antimercury supplements to protect myself?" I am not very comfortable in approving of loading the body with mercury at one end and trying at the same time to get rid of it at the other. On the other hand, in this context a critical question has been raised by medical nutritionists. Should we not worry only about those who are sensitive to mercury? Not all patients are. Others are exquisitely sensitive, reacting to a mercury patch test with symptoms so violent that some dentists will no longer use the test. Should these be the only patients tested for mercury retention, and treated if it is found? The assumption here would be that all the others have managed to cope with the mercury by one body process or another, or by a happy choice of diet. But when I discussed this subject with dentists who have been engaged in research on the amalgam problem, one of the replies was, "What do you want to do—wait until the patient has a heart attack?"

Science always brings up more questions than are answered. In the matter of mercury poisoning from amalgam, the unanswered questions are clearly significant and troublesome. I personally believe that when scientists fall out, the only possible choice for the public is the pathway of safety.

Let me emphasize the relevance of this discussion in a text on hypoglycemia. Many of the symptoms of hypoglycemia are duplicated or intensified by mercury poisoning. The diet that produces or worsens hypoglycemia is the diet that produces tooth decay, the need for amalgam, and the risk of mercury poisoning. The lesson in prevention is obvious.

# 12. New Findings in Diet for Diabetics and Hypoglycemics

As fiber is used to help hypoglycemics (see page 171), so is it useful to diabetics. A high fiber intake is beneficial to diabetics, with one proviso: they must choose sources to which they are not allergic. The average diabetic does not consider himself a victim of allergy. He is serenely unaware that an allergic reaction to a food can significantly elevate his blood sugar, and that this is true whether the food is a sugar, starch, protein, or fat.

He is also unaware of what is called "the glycemic index," a term that requires careful explanation, beginning with a review of medical practices that remain unaltered, despite this new information. For many years, diabetic clinics and diabetologists have supplied their patients with lists of food exchanges. Essentially, these lists are based upon a simple and apparently justifiable premise: if you, the diabetic, do not feel like eating spaghetti, you can take a calorie-equivalent portion of carbohydrate from any other food. Thus you might substitute rice, baked potato, or bread for the spaghetti, in portions yielding approximately the same number of calories from starch. For many years, we in the avant-garde movement of nutrition have pointed out that carbohydrate is carbohydrate, but different foods in that family, even in the same portions, do not have the same effects on blood sugar. Wheat, for example, will raise blood sugar much more than an equivalent portion of rice. We pressured the diabetic establishment to recognize that what is important is not equivalence in calories but equivalence in biological effects. To all this they turned a deaf ear and to this day have not adequately acted on the information, even though it has been amply authenticated.

Not only do identical portions of different carbohydrates have different effects on blood sugar, but the manner in which the food is prepared and the amount of fiber accompanying it will alter the results in terms of blood sugar. As I noted earlier, a dry baked potato, minus the skin, has the same effect as sugar. Taken with fat, it acts like starch, meaning slower absorption and less impact on blood sugar level. A firm rice pudding acts on blood sugar like a starch. A loose portion of rice, prepared as a slurry in plenty of liquid, will act like sugar. There is also no easily recognized difference between the blood sugar effects of simple and complex carbohydrates. Some of the simple sugars cause a slow and moderate rise in the levels of blood sugar, while some of the starches elevate the blood sugar quickly and sharply.

For these reasons, I present a glycemic index, which should be useful to both diabetics and hypoglycemics. The foods and numerical ratings given are those that have been researched at present. The higher the index number of the food, the greater the metabolic difficulty with it. The lower the number, the more satisfactory the food. The glycemic index is affected by the manner of the food's preparation and by the accompanying foods eaten.

*The sugars* do not act alike. Fructose, or fruit sugar, while it is not the perfect food for hypoglycemics and diabetics, as has been described, does enter the blood more slowly. It is also metabolized more slowly, since the body converts it into glucose, and the conversion takes time. This does not mean that the eulogies of fructose as safe for everybody are justified, for there are both hypoglycemics and diabetics who react diversely to substantial intake of fructose. On the glycemic index, fructose rates a 20. Sucrose, or white sugar, is rated at 59. Honey, so long a favorite with the health-minded, ranks as 87—not astonishing, since honey is merely predigested sugar. And glucose, as you might anticipate, rates 100, least desirable of all forms of sugars for the hypoglycemic and diabetic.

*The grains* hold some surprises. Whole wheat spaghetti has the lowest number for the grains in the glycemic index: 42. Ordinary spaghetti, 50. Sweet corn, though it supplies fiber is 59. Brown rice, 68 (which its fiber content would seem to belie). White bread is slightly worse than white sugar with a 69, but the surprise comes with whole wheat bread—72. White rice ends the list, also 72.

*The breakfast cereals* are generally quickly absorbed. Oatmeal ranks at 49; all bran at 51; Swiss muesli, 66. Shredded wheat is unexpectedly 67, and cornflakes, the best-selling dry cereal, is the worst: 80. The ranking of the bran cereal probably would be better if the cereal were

free of added sugar, but most such cereals are sweetened by the manufacturer.

*The fruits* give you an idea of the impact of food processing. Very few
of us sit down and eat a half dozen apples, but it is easy to drink the
equivalent of that number in the form of juice. Apples, whole, are
ranked at a 39 in the glycemic index, but apple juice is much higher.
Oranges are 40; orange juice, 46. (It is obvious that consuming the
whole fruit conveys some dividends, including exercise for your teeth
and gums.) Bananas rank 62, although there are no data to indicate
whether fully ripe bananas, which are pure sugar, or partially ripe
bananas, which are starch, were tested. Raisins, as you might anticipate, rank 64.

Among *the root vegetables*, sweet potatoes are the lowest, only 48.
Yams come in at 51, and beets at 64. Note the difference in the next
two figures: white potatoes rank 70, but instant mashed potatoes climb
to an undesirable 80. Carrots rank 92—they are comparatively rich in
sugar; and parsnips are 97, which is a surprise.

In *the dairy products*, skim milk is the most slowly absorbed: 32.
Whole milk, as one might expect from its fat content, comes off better:
34. Ice cream, again because of its fat content, is 36. Yogurt also ranks
36, but I do not know whether high-fat or low-fat yogurt was tested.
The difference might be significant, and the yogurt with a normal fat
content more desirable.

Among *the peas and beans*, dry, canned, and frozen, soybeans have
the most desirable ranking: 15. Lentils and kidney beans are identical
in the glycemic index: 29. Black-eyed peas, 33. Chick-peas and lima
beans rank alike: 36. Canned baked beans, 40 (which may be a result of
the sugar frequently added to this product). Frozen peas rank last, with
a dismal 51.

Peanuts are obviously a good choice for the hypoglycemic and the
diabetic, with a ranking of only 13. Sponge cake is an invitation to
trouble: 46. Potato chips more so, with a 51. If you want a comparison
with the obvious: a candy bar ranks 68.

This generalization can be made: the more highly processed the food
is, the more quickly it may raise the blood sugar. This is undesirable not
only for a diabetic, but for a hypoglycemic as well, who by definition
overreacts to blood sugar when it rises too suddenly.

The manner in which a food is cooked or processed, the amount of fiber in the food, the methods of cooking and processing, and the accompanying types of foods appear to be factors in the blood sugar response. Years of study will be necessary to evaluate the influence of these variables.

# 13. Grocery Shopping Contaminated with Biological Sanity

If you have read this far, it may be that this book has persuaded you that it is common sense to be as intelligent in selecting food as you presumably are in seeking treatment to offset what your present diet has done to you. If that is the case, please accept an invitation to let the nutritionist accompany you to the supermarket, where you will observe his selections and, as important, his rejections, and ponder the reasons for both. As you do so, remember that the American Establishment will not approve of this chaperoned shopping expedition, for it frowns on rejection of *any* of its food products, the premise being that an indiscriminately selected, mixed diet guarantees optimal nutrition, all edibles being highly desirable. This is based on the ancient doctrine that it is best to ignore ugly facts that interfere with beautiful theories—or soaring profits.

*Snack foods:* The nutritionist races through this department so fast that there is but enough time for you to read one label so that you may realize that these snacks are predominantly overprocessed carbohydrates, lacking essential vitamins and minerals. (It is an interesting quirk of the law that vitamin enrichment, required for white bread, is optional in sweetened baked products, though sugar raises vitamin requirements!) The snack foods are cleverly packaged, of course, but they are loaded with preservatives and antioxidants. The nutritionist buys whole wheat and whole rye crackers and potato chips. The chips are made with potatoes, salt, and vegetable oil. A competitive brand, rejected, is dosed with butyl-hydroxy-anisole (BHA), butyl-hydroxy-toluene (BHT), and, perhaps, propyl-gallate. Children like potato chips, and the younger the child, the less equipped he is to metabolize (break down) these chemicals, with which his body (and yours) possesses no physiological experience. The propagandists for the processed-food industry sometimes use the sophistry of pointing out that all food is essentially a combination of chemicals. So why object to a few more? Apart from the obvious fact that our bodies are equipped to deal with (and profit by) chemicals indigenous to food, one is entitled to carry the argument through to its logical extreme and justify a little arsenic for seasoning.

With honey, onion dip, or a good cheese, the whole grain crackers make a delightful and sustaining snack. In some stores you will find brown rice crackers. These are equally desirable.

*Produce:* One would think that shopping for fruits and vegetables would have a built-in fail-safe factor, and for the most part that is true. However, the nutritionist is unhappy about the bleaching of endive (and, in the past, celery), for color in these foods is associated with pigment-bearing minerals and vitamins, and bleaching subtracts values. He also deplores the domination of salad recipes by head lettuce, perhaps the lowest of all salad greens in nutrient values. He buys fenuche, Boston lettuce, romaine, chicory, escarole, Chinese cabbage (using the outer green leaves in salad), and tender beet greens (for salad and cooking). He uses tomatoes, cabbage, avocado, watercress, chives, parsley, scallions, and onions, and winds up with varied and succulent salads. He also varies the dressings, keeping a weather eye peeled for the ubiquitous BHT additive, which appears in many of these products.

*Meats, fowl, fish:* Patronize the butcher; cut down on visits to the baker. Buy more fish, which is good, high-quality protein and inexpensive. Inspect fish carefully, for it is amazing how a bath in brine and ice will make aged fish seem youthful. While insecticide residues have been found in meat, they have also appeared in deep-sea fish caught sixty miles off shore. Man can't spray the ocean, but he can spray wholesale fish markets.

Let me repeat the admonition that in buying meat, you must drop the assumption that steak, rib roast, and filet mignon are the principal parts of the animal. Actually, many "less desirable" cuts of meat are equally nutritious, flavorful, and, if properly tenderized and cooked, tender. Marination of meat in wine or use of papaya tenderizers are among acceptable ways in which to make block chuck cuts tender and succulent. Such meats are actually chosen by the gourmet in preference to the T-bone steaks, sirloins, and porterhouse cuts. Don't pass by beef plate, beef neck, shin, lungs, heart, sweetbread, brains, kidney, and liver. Don't avoid pork. Just cook it properly for safety; it is a very nutritious meat. The organ meats of all species are particularly nutritious foods, and there is really no unwritten law that says that liver can be served only once a week. If you don't know how to prepare such cuts and organ meats in varied ways, consult Adelle Davis' *Let's Cook It Right* or *The Carlton Fredericks Cookbook for Good Nutrition.*

Delicatessen meats are expensive in terms of the amount of protein they supply. (Actually, in those terms, bologna is more costly than sirloin steak.) Many of these products are garnished with forms of sugar, including dextrose, sucrose, or corn syrup. Virtually all contain nitrates (see note, page 163), which offer gratuitous danger. When they don't contain nitrates, they are preserved with (usually, too much) salt.

Never buy meats or fish conspicuously lower in price than similar buys at other markets. Meat prices at wholesale level are remarkably stable, so much so that a chain buying millions of dollars of meat may enjoy but a few cents price advantage over the neighborhood butcher shop. Unless the supermarket is taking a loss to bring traffic into the store, which is a common practice, be wary of sales which are over-dramatic. It's amazing how a "bargain" corn beef, twenty cents per pound cheaper than average, can shrink to nothing in cooking, indicating that a larcenous butcher used the brine hypo to an illegal extent. With regard to the beautifying effects of salt and ice on fish, it is best not to buy fresh seafood products on Mondays unless you know that the store received a delivery on that day. (The same point applies to salad greens that may have been stored over a long weekend. In any case, you should not buy produce displayed without refrigeration. This applies to eggs, too; they age unbelievably at room temperature—even in no more than twenty-four hours.)

The nutritionist is not enthusiastic about chicken (or eggs) produced by fowl that never touch the ground, for this is the condition of the modern chicken-egg factory. The ration is supposed to be "scientific," promoting fantastically rapid growth in the chicks. Yet that rapid growth has been accompanied by epidemics of hemorrhagic disease, which have wiped out entire flocks, indicating that the diet does not supply adequate amounts of unknown nutrients needed for maximum fowl health. Chicken, too, is costly: when the dressed bird is selling at $.69 per pound, the actual cost of the meat may reach $1.50 per pound. With the reservation, then, that the chicken of yesteryear may have been better nutrition—and certainly had better flavor—fowl is a recommended buy when prices are down. (And for those who think that the chicken diet, being the product of modern science, must be superb, please remember that the diet for fingerling trout, likewise a scientific triumph, decimated virtually all the fish—with cancer!)

*Beverages:* In view of what you have read concerning the direct role of caffeine in coffee and cola drinks in causing and aggravating hypoglycemia, one would anticipate that the nutritionist would vote in favor of the decaffeinated coffees. However, it's obvious that one person's allergy to strawberries does not force you to excommunicate the fruit, and those who tolerate coffee certainly will not suffer if they consume a cup or two daily. If one wishes to be an alarmist, one can find something potentially hazardous in a majority of foods; coffee, for instance, by virtue of the roasting process, could conceivably contain carcinogenic (cancer-causing) substances, but the reality of the situation is that millions of Americans drink billions of cups of the beverage without being decimated by cancer. The nutritionist does not view with alarm everything you enjoy, and if coffee does not overstimulate you, and if you do not have hypoglycemia or a tendency toward it, or fibrocystic breast disease, this favorite beverage can hold its place in your nutritional scheme of things. Not so with the cola beverages. Their sugar content is absurd. Their acidity is shocking, one of them having as much as vinegar, which would make it no boon to teeth, and a bottle contains a quantity of caffeine equivalent to over one-fourth of a cup of coffee. The sugarless cola beverage still supplies caffeine, and the nutritionist, although the artificial sweeteners have been declared safe,* sees no point in abusing them as you have abused sugar.

Juices require consumer caution. The shelves are packed with "juice drinks," labeled so as to be characterized as "juices" in the consumer's mind. These concoctions represent, usually, a blend of a little fruit juice, much water and sugar, a dollop of citric acid, and, sometimes, a little added Vitamin C. The buyer conscious of good nutrition will buy *juices*, and that does not mean the synthetic breakfast "juice-like" drinks that combine Vitamin C, artificial flavor, artificial color, and

---

* Artificial sweeteners presently available may be safe, in reasonable quantities, for the average person, but they should not be used, even in small amounts, by pregnant women. Allergic individuals should be tested for tolerance of them.

much sugar. There are many nutrients in fruits that are not found in these masqueraders, and contrary to what the public has been told, there *is* a difference in the natural carbohydrates of foods—juices, in this case—and the processed sugar used in the imitation drinks.

Coffee-like beverages—usually based on roasted wheat—are harmless, but they present a hazard to those with peptic ulcer, for their ability to evoke acid production is surprisingly close to that of coffee itself.

*Dairy foods:* Observe the dating system used on milk and cream cartons in your store. It is useful to know when milk, cream, skim milk, and buttermilk were delivered and should be sold by.

The nutritionist buys yogurt, but without the added jams and preserves. Add your own fruit, if you desire, and escape the unbelievable amount of sugar added to the jam-laden flavored yogurts. Contrary to propaganda aimed at "food faddists," there *is* a difference in the biological effects of yogurt as compared with sweet milk products. Animals fed this food live longer and have more resistance to infections. The food is also useful in restoring bacterial flora of the intestinal tract to normal after it has been decimated by antibiotics.

Butter versus margarine? There is no "versus." Buy butter, and depend on the vegetable oils for unsaturated fat. As indicated earlier, the partially hydrogenated fats, used in hundreds of foods, are potentially dangerous, causing or aggravating the symptoms of many diseases. (This is why margarine has been deleted from the recipes and menus of this revised edition of the book.)

If your budget means anything, do not buy liquid skim milk. Buy powdered nonfat milk, which offers exactly the same food values at a much lower price. If you're really pinched for funds, serve 1¼ ounces of butter for each quart of reconstituted nonfat milk you serve the family, and they will get the equivalent of whole milk at about half the price. The nonfat milk powder is most useful, too, in fortifying cereals, cakes, muffins, and pancakes, as well as home-baked bread, with larger amounts of fine milk protein and calcium. It also improves their texture and flavor.

Watch the additives in synthetic cream! If you are a Jew who eats only kosher foods, avoid those which contain "calcium caseinate," for casein is always a milk product. (The manufacturers have decided, however, that this fact doesn't stop them from calling these products "nondairy.")

Brown and white eggs are nutritionally equal. In choosing among small, medium, and large eggs, remember that these terms signify weights: 18, 21, and 24 ounces to the dozen. The price difference should be proportionate; if it isn't, choose the better bargain. There are nutritionists who find today's egg, with its thin shell and flat flavor, to be a commentary on modern "egg factory" methods of feeding the birds. If you agree, try to buy "organic" eggs. You will know by the strength of the shell that the hens have been fed a good diet, which will be reflected in the egg's flavor, too. The theory that a fertilized egg is better nutrition is only theory; there is no convincing evidence to buttress it, although, among the better-known egg experts, at least one holds it to be true.

Ice cream is 16 percent sugar, which is no boon to the pancreas. A total of 58 additives—added by the manufacturer or by way of the components of the recipe—was counted in one brand. Use ice cream with discretion, unless you're hypoglycemic, in which case, avoid it. The "diabetic" ice creams are often sheer fraud, supplying almost as many calories from carbohydrates as do the "regular" brands. The ices are suspect, many of them containing artificial color and flavor—both of which you can manage to do without.

*Syrups:* Strictly speaking, maple syrup is sugar of several types, plus a small mineral content, but that is more than is provided by the imitations. One maple syrup producer has been unwilling to label his product as "pure maple syrup" ever since the FDA allowed the industry to use formaldehyde to keep the sap holes free of bacteria, which, of course, introduced a formaldehyde content (five parts per million) in the syrup. Previously, the industry had legally used chlorine bleach, which disappeared in the processing, for this purpose. At least one producer of an imitation maple syrup is claiming a "buttery" flavor, which reflects no butter content at all. Dark molasses remains a good choice, or blackstrap that has been cleaned for human consumption. The latter supplies fifteen times as much iron and much more calcium than ordinary molasses and a surprising assortment of vitamins, as well.

*Pancake and cake mixes:* Sugar and more sugar, with a full load of additives, including preservatives, artificial colors, artificial flavors, and, frequently, partially hydrogenated fats. Much saner recipes will be found in health-food store products, but even there you must read labels carefully.

*Frozen and canned vegetables and fruits:* The frozen varieties have an advantage over the canned. Freezing does not ordinarily alter the food, but preserves it as it was when processed—and the processing is frequently done right at the site of production of the crop. The canned food is actually cooked, for safety; and the variety chosen and the degree of ripeness allowable is determined by the consideration that heat will be applied. Some varieties and certain stages of ripeness must therefore be avoided, if the food is to be canned, to prevent mush being the end product in the container. Losses of vitamins do occur in canning—no greater, certainly, than you would encounter in home preparation—and the large canning companies maintain quality control departments that exclude what you cannot avoid in fresh produce: crops too heavily laden with insecticide residue. (The Heinz Company once discarded tens of thousands of dollars' worth of vegetables intended for packing for baby food because there was too much insecticide.) Frozen foods have been reported to suffer a significant loss of Vitamin K. In spite of all these observations, these foods are still good nutrition, with but one reservation: both canned and frozen fruits are insanely saturated with sugar. It is encouraging, however, to note that at least two pineapple packers discovered that self-juice packing makes for a much better, more palatable product than the syrup-laden fruit they formerly promoted.

The frozen prepared dinners may be useful in an emergency, but the large majority of them shortchange you on protein, the most expensive ingredient. This can be compensated for by serving cheese for dessert, by baking nonfat milk into a dessert recipe, and by using similar devices. Many convenience foods are filled with additives—read labels!

*Baby foods:* A tribute was paid, two paragraphs back, to the integrity of a baby food manufacturer. Now a criticism is in order: there is too much sugar in baby fruits. It is a pathway to the excessive appetite for sweets that leads many children into tooth decay and, perhaps, in later life, into hypoglycemia. There is also something less than reassuring in "liver soup" that contains less than 6 percent liver! Buy baby foods selectively—as carefully as, after this journey, you buy your own food.

*Dog food:* Frequently, in dog food, there is better nutrition than in food packed for human consumption by the same manufacturers. Choose those made from meat. After all, the dog is a carnivorous animal. The dog profits from organ meats, just as people do.

*Cereals:* It is heartening to know that the boxes of cereals that go into space with the astronauts are said to be made from packaging materials which themselves are edible. It is time that something nutritious went into some of these cereals! The "puffed" or exploded cereals have not only been degerminated, with resultant loss of the natural Vitamin B Complex, but their protein values are denatured by the process. The flaked cereals, because of their flake form, are subjected to much heat in processing, with the result that you will find whole wheat cereals that are vitamin-enriched—an enrichment needed, ordinarily, only by cereals that have lost significant percentages of their vitamin content. Many of the cereals are pre-sugared by the manufacturer, the premise being, I suppose, that anyone who eats food of this kind will obviously be too weak to lift his own sugar spoon. Some cereals actually contain candy and should be sold in the candy department, rather than being masqueraded as foods. A portion of cereal weighs but one ounce; this is equivalent to a slice of bread, yet the advertising is so compelling that some mothers consider a portion of such a food a breakfast suitable for a schoolchild. Buy whole grain cereals, whole wheat, particularly. Buy wheat germ in vacuum-packed jars, and use it as a cereal and to fortify all other cereals—a spoonful to a portion. Make no distinction between hot and cold cereals; the nutritional value is not determined by cooking or lack of it. Some hot cereals are poor food, some dry cereals are good nutrition. A few hot cereals of the highly processed types are now fortified with wheat germ by the manufacturers. Oatmeal remains a good buy, and the quick cooking type is acceptable. For all their ingenuity, the processors have never come up with a technique of nutritionally wrecking oats as they have wrecked corn, rice, and wheat. Avoid the cereals that offer a "full vitamin ration" in the daily portion. Such supplements are never as well balanced as those in capsules and syrups, which also offer the advantage of providing a natural source of the entire Vitamin B Complex.

*Cooking oils:* Cottonseed oil has so much Vitamin E in it that the manufacturers do not find it necessary to add antioxidants. Other oils are garnished with BHT, BHA, and other additives. Sesame oil is a good choice, as is safflower oil when the additives are not used. Wheat germ oil is an excellent addition to salad oil, but is not to be used for cooking. It brings up both the Vitamin E and the polyunsaturated fat ration.

*Breads:* The fine value of all grain germs—wheat germ, corn germ, etc.—is in itself voluble criticism of the rape of the grain represented by white bread, rye bread (which has more white wheat flour than rye, and the rye is also overprocessed), and cracked wheat bread (which is 85 percent white flour). Pumpernickel is essentially a fermented rye bread with all the sins of the latter, plus an artificial suntan derived from burned sugar. The phrase "caramel color added" reveals the over-processed bread, for real pumpernickel, the peasant bread, is whole rye bread and requires no added color. Whole rye bread is excellent nutrition and most palatable, which explains why it is so difficult to track down and buy. Corn sticks and muffins made from degerminated corn have lost important nutritional values and grow brick hard in hours. Why is a whole corn muffin impossible to locate? Bake them at home, and when you buy cornmeal, stay away from the degerminated kind! One must read labels carefully. At least one manufacturer tried to hide the fact that the product was degerminated by stating that "We have removed the oils that tend to cause rancidity." The oils referred to are those in the germ, and you buy them back as corn oil.

Bagels are boiled before they are baked, the assumption being that any nutrients that escape the milling will succumb to drowning. The same is true of pretzels.

Occasionally, one will find a white bread that has been fortified with wheat germ. This is an excellent compromise, although not so satisfactory as whole wheat bread.

Storebought cakes, Danish pastry, doughnuts, and cookies are an excellent route to diabetes or hypoglycemia, tooth decay, hemorrhoids, and irregularity. Bake your own.

You have now completed your supermarket journey. Don't let the mass of details subtract from your determination to feed yourself and your family well. It will all shortly become reflex, except for the ever-renewed joy of seeing your efforts contribute to heightened well-being for you and yours, and for the knowledge that you are influencing the destiny of children as yet unconceived, as yet unborn.

## Supplements to the Hypoglycemia Diet

Allergy may restrict your use of dietary supplements, and it is worth knowing that a mixture of amino acids, in the free form, placed under the tongue, may relieve many of the cerebral symptoms of allergy. Likewise, combined use of Vitamin C and Vitamin B6, taken simultaneously, may relieve allergy symptoms. When allergy has been prolonged and severe, there may be elevation of histamine in the tissues, which can slowly be reduced with supplements of calcium and methionine. Vitamin C itself is an efficient antihistamine, and relieves some allergy symptoms. Consult your medical nutritionist. If you need referral to such a practitioner, consult Appendix I, "Resources for Nutritional Counseling," page 233.

Where tolerance permits, brewer's yeast (not torula yeast) and dessicated liver, in tablets and capsules, are useful sources of the Vitamin B Complex in its natural, whole form. Wheat germ, formerly recommended for this purpose, may be contaminated with EDB, and should be avoided until the problem is solved.

The minimum supplement for hypoglycemics is a multiple vitamin, multiple mineral, and a separate Vitamin B Complex concentrate, taken in label dosage. The Vitamin B Complex chosen should supply at least 1000 mgs. of choline and 500 mgs. of inositol. Many products don't, but these factors may be purchased separately. They are important to liver function and thereby to hypoglycemics.

The chromium glucose-tolerance factor, derived from yeast, should not be used in the metallic chromium form, which must be converted to the factor by the body; because you are hypoglycemic, your conversion may be faulty. Your health-food store is familiar with such products.

All this is dietary insurance, and applying it is not optional but mandatory. Recovery from an illness—and certainly low blood sugar is one—requires higher intake of essential nutrients than the dietary supply.

## Food Additives: Bane or Benefit?

While the Food and Drug Administration of the United States government has spent millions of dollars in regulating the vitamin industry—to the point where it has been accused of trying to destroy over-the-counter sales of vitamin supplements—it has been curiously lenient in its policies toward food additives. Butyl-hydroxy-toluene is an excellent case in point. This chemical was originally used as an antioxidant for color motion picture film. It then emerged as an ingredient in everything from cereals to chewing gum, from sausages to salad oil.

Australian investigators charged that BHT was teratogenic (interfering with normal development of the embryo.) Pregnant animals fed the chemical bore young with a shocking incidence of complete absence of eyes. Others found that the antioxidant depressed the activity of three important blood enzymes, caused enlargement of the liver, and was retained in the organism long enough to indicate that the body was having difficulty in metabolizing (breaking down) the material into less toxic substances.

A consumer research group queried the FDA concerning the papers and the research on which they based acceptance of BHT as a food ingredient. The astonishing reply was that the papers were "secret" (or words to that effect). When this was publicized, the agency grudgingly released the scientific reports. It turned out that there were only two, both written by the staff of the manufacturers of BHT!

The World Health Organization of the United Nations warned that BHT should not be fed to babies. The British Ministry of Food considered banning it, but took no action. You are still swallowing it. It appears on the label in its own right—as butyl-hydroxy-toluene, as BHT, or disguised as "freshness preserver" or "oxygen interceptor." I don't care to swallow it, or to give it to children.

The story of Red #4 is equally striking. The FDA licensed the use of this coal-tar dye in food and then later proposed to ban it. Tests had revealed it to be carcinogenic (cancer-producing) in dogs. At this point, the pharmaceutical industry, which uses it on pills, protested. They asked for a "few years'" delay in the ban, pleading that they, too, were testing and needed time to complete the research. The ban was rescinded. You continued to ingest Red #4 for a relatively long time. Then Red #2 was substituted, in lipsticks, vitamin pills, and even in white cake icing and soda pop, though the evidence shows that it, too, is unacceptably dangerous.

Nordihydroguaiaretic acid (NDGA) has a more reassuring history. The FDA took time off from castigating vitamin users as food faddists and licensed the use of this additive in food. Canadian toxicological studies indicted it as dangerous. The FDA was forced, apparently, to follow the lead of its counterpart in Canada, the Food and Drug Directorate, and withdraw the licensing of the material. Yet in March 1968, the U.S. Department of Agriculture, a year after the Canadian report, licensed NDGA for use in dry sausage, along with other antioxidants!

Many additives are in use without formal testing, being GRAS ("generally regarded as safe") because of many years of use. This assurance is no assurance at all. One need only remember, if evidence is needed to denigrate the validity of this term, the history of coumarin, a vanilla substitute, which, after many years of use as a food additive "generally regarded as safe," was found to produce tumors in animals. The story of "butter-yellow," a food coloring material, is another case in point. We swallowed it in foods for more than twenty years after Germany banned it as a cancer-producing material.

A crusade against food additives generically would be folly. Certainly, though, one does not invite toxicity or cancer by the additives one does not ingest, and the story of BHT, NDGA, coumarin, and butter-yellow would suggest that, all other factors being equal, it is more sensible to buy the foods least heavily laden with these triumphs of modern food technology. Then you need have no apprehensions when, one day, you pick up your morning paper and read that a GRAS additive has suddenly been found to be teratogenic, carcinogenic, or merely somewhat poisonous.

# Appendixes

## I. RESOURCES FOR NUTRITIONAL COUNSELING

Though all physicians, generally, dispense diets and advice for use (or nonuse) of dietary supplements, medical nutritionists have special skills in this area. You can secure referral to such an expert by sending $3.00 to the International Academy of Preventive Medicine, 34 Corporate Woods, Suite 469, 10950 Grandview, Overland Park, Kansas 66210. You will receive its national directory of medical nutritionists. Be sure to note each doctor's specialization. It will do you no good to consult a nutritional proctologist if the trouble is in your ears (or your blood sugar). Another society with similar membership is the International College of Applied Nutrition, P.O. Box 386, La Habra, California 90631. Please note that national membership doesn't mean there'll be a practitioner around the corner. You may have to travel for the help you need.

If you are seeking orthomolecular psychiatry, which emphasizes therapy in the treatment of schizophrenia, depression, manic-depressive disorders, autism, mental retardation, learning disabilities, senility, hyperactivity, hypoglycemia, and cerebral allergies, contact the Academy of Orthomolecular Psychiatry, 1691 Northern Boulevard, Manhasset, Long Island, New York 11030. At the same address is the North Nassau Mental Health Center, which directly treats such patients.

The Princeton Brain Bio Center, a pioneering facility for biochemical treatment of mental and emotional disorders, is at 862 Route 518, Skillman, New Jersey 08558.

Guidance for psychotic, autistic, and learning-disabled children is available through the Institute for Child Behavior Research, 5147

Adams Avenue, San Diego, California 92116, which gives parents access to both orthomolecular and psychotherapeutic help for children.

For alcoholism, there is a successful treatment combining nutritional and psychiatric therapies available at Health Recovery Associates, 3255 Hennepin Avenue South, Minneapolis, Minnesota 55408.

For allergists who are aware that hypoglycemia triggers or worsens allergy, that food allergy does exist, and that neutralizing techniques are sometimes therapeutic, write to the Society for Clinical Ecology, Robert Collier, MD, Secretary-Treasurer, 4045 Wadsworth Boulevard, P.O. Box 16106, Denver, Colorado 80216.

# II. TESTS RELATED TO HYPOGLYCEMIA

## Self-Test for Low Blood Sugar (Hypoglycemia)

Try this test yourself. Simply multiply each "yes" answer in the first column by three; each "yes" in the second column by two. Add the two totals and if the score is over 58—see your doctor! You may have a dangerous sugar imbalance—hypoglycemia—that may be totally responsible for a wide variety of ills hitherto believed to be emotionally or psychologically based.

|                                     | I |                              | II |
|-------------------------------------|---|------------------------------|----|
| Nervousness                         |   | Exhaustion                   |    |
| Irritability                        |   | Faintness, tremors,          |    |
| Depression                          |   |   cold sweats, weak          |    |
| Forgetfulness                       |   |   spells                     |    |
| Insomnia (awakening in              |   | Vertigo                      |    |
|   the small hours, un-              |   | Drowsiness                   |    |
|   able to return to sleep)          |   | Headaches                    |    |
| Constant worrying                   |   | Chronic indigestion          |    |
| Mental confusion                    |   | Internal trembling           |    |
| Unsocial, antisocial,               |   | Palpitation of the heart     |    |
|   asocial behavior                  |   | Rapid pulse                  |    |
| Unprovoked crying spells            |   | Muscle pain                  |    |
| Indecisiveness                      |   | Numbness                     |    |
| Lack of sexual drive                |   | Allergies                    |    |
|   (women)                           |   | Incoordination               |    |

| I | | II | |
|---|---|---|---|
| Impotence | _____ | Leg Cramps | _____ |
| Night terrors, night-mares | _____ | Blurred vision | _____ |
| Phobias, fears | _____ | Twitching, jerking, cramping of leg muscles | _____ |
| Suicidal thoughts | _____ | Itching and crawling sensations on skin | _____ |
| Restlessness | _____ | Gasping for breath | _____ |
| Nervous breakdowns | _____ | Smothering spells | _____ |
| | | Staggering | _____ |
| | | Unconsciousness | _____ |
| | | Rheumatoid arthritis | _____ |
| | | Neurodermatitis | _____ |
| | | Lack of appetite | _____ |
| | | Compulsive craving for sweets, colas, coffee, tea | _____ |
| | | Joint pains | _____ |
| | | Abdominal spasms | _____ |
| | | Obesity | _____ |
| | | Underweight | _____ |
| | | Compulsive drinking of alcoholic beverages | _____ |

## The Pulse Test

Many years ago, Dr. Arthur Coca discovered that an acceleration of the pulse is a very common reaction in allergic people exposed to foods, drugs, and chemicals to which they are sensitive. The pulse test is not infallible—for reasons which will be explained—but frequently it is surprisingly accurate.

Before beginning the test, smokers must stop smoking, because once again tobacco sensitivity can distort the results of the test. If you are curious about your possible sensitivity to tobacco, that can be tested after you have gone through the foods.

The first thing you must learn to do is to count your own pulse—how many times your heart beats per minute. Do not count the beats for fifteen seconds and multiply by four, because you may introduce enough inaccuracy to invalidate the test.

You then keep a record of your pulse rate, with fourteen separate recordings daily, for at least two days before the test. Record your one-minute pulse count on awakening in the morning, before any activity. Do it again immediately before you eat. Repeat for each meal. Also take your pulse three times, every thirty minutes, for an hour and a half after meals. Finally, take your pulse before going to sleep.

Snacks are considered meals and should be charted, too, with the times at which you ate them. Your pulse record before the snack and three times subsequently, at intervals of a half hour, is again necessary.

It is not only necessary to make a record of your pulse counts on these occasions, but also to make one of your menus. Please remember that some foods contain many ingredients, and it is possible that you are sensitive to one or more of them. You therefore must read labels, and in the record of the foods you eat at each meal, each ingredient should be listed.

These records supply a baseline. Knowing your pulse characteristics enables you after testing to determine if there has been a variation which may be significant in terms of allergy. The recordings of your pulse prior to testing tell you the lowest rate of your pulse during the day, the highest, and your pulse differential, which is the difference between those two rates.

Pulse rates tend to be pretty uniform for each individual, but don't forget that there are stress factors, independent of allergy, which can change the rate. If you have been living alone and suddenly find yourself eating breakfast with an attractive stranger of the opposite sex, your pulse reading may be extremely deceptive. Exercise, of course, will also change it. The lowest pulse rate usually occurs before you leave your bed in the morning. Even this is subject to qualification if you happen to be intolerant of your pillow stuffing, or the dust in your mattress, or, possibly, something you consumed the day before. In that case, your initial pulse on awakening, the first day, may well be deceptive— higher than it will be later in the week.

These are the numbers that will be meaningful:

1. If your pulse rises more than 12 beats during any single day, the chance is that you are sensitive to something you ate that particular day. If your pulse rises more than 16 beats, the sensitivity is almost certain. Conversely, if your pulse does not rise more than 12 beats on

any of the days when you are establishing the baseline, it is probable that your meals were not disturbing you on those days.

2. Experience shows that an unusual increase in your characteristic pulse rate on any single occasion points to a strong probability of a sensitivity reaction (assuming that you don't have a bad case of sunburn, an attractive stranger across the table, or a session of violent exercise).

Having established the characteristics of your pulse rate, you are now ready to spend two days pinning down possible allergies by testing foods individually.

You begin by recording your awakening pulse, as you did before. For the rest of the day, you eat on the hour, a different food each time. Just before eating, record your pulse, and then record it again a half hour after eating. If after eating a food your pulse goes up as described above, you must wait until it returns to its normal rate before you go on to another test. Sometimes a reaction to a food to which you are sensitive can last for a few hours. There may also be variations in your pulse in which there is a higher rate after eating a food, then a drop, and then an increase again, and this may happen several times before the pulse returns to its normal pattern. After any increase in the pulse rate, you must allow it to go back to and remain normal for at least an hour before testing the next food. Otherwise, you will not know which food was responsible for your reaction.

Staying away from a food may allow the body to build defenses. Therefore, if you test a food that you have not consumed for some weeks, there may be no pulse reaction. The test should be repeated two or three days later if it involves something that you eat infrequently.

There is one disturbing factor in evaluating foods by the pulse rate method: some individuals are so allergic that unknowing and continued exposure to their sensitizing agents will give them a constant pulse rate above 84. For them, the pulse test is not useful, although the rate suggests the need for testing by other means for sensitivity to food or other factors in the environment.

And now for smokers: when you have pinned down your pulse reactions and thereby your sensitivities to foods (and, incidentally, to chemicals, inhalants, and the gas from your stove), you are ready to go back to smoking. If you also want to know if you are sensitive to tobacco, there is a simple index: your pulse will usually betray your intolerance for tobacco within fifteen minutes from the time you smoke your first cigarette.

## Kinesiological Testing

This method of testing for food and chemical sensitivities is based on a sound observation which, nonetheless, the public finds unbelievable. Intolerance, sensitivity, or allergy to a food, drug, chemical, or inhalant, is indicated by a significant loss of strength in the muscle after exposure. Because of the skepticism of the public and, indeed, of a large percentage of the professional community, I have not frequently recommended self-testing kinesiologically for allergy and intolerance.

To give you an idea of a simplified application of kinesiology, hold your arm to the side with the palm down. Have the person testing you place one pinkie on your wrist and his other hand on your shoulder on the same side. Push against his finger. At the same time, he should push down firmly, as if trying to make your arm drop. This is not a wrestling match; it is merely a means of establishing some measure of your muscle tone.

You are now ready to test a food to determine specifically if it is capable of causing disturbances of brain chemistry. Briefly chew a small amount of food, then place it under your tongue. If you are testing a liquid, hold it in your mouth for a moment to let it mix with saliva, then hold it beneath your tongue. Please note that the food is not to be swallowed. Swallowing it may induce a systemic reaction which may be of long duration and will thereby interfere with the accuracy of the testing.

Wait about two minutes, and then have your partner retest the muscle, exactly as it was done before. If your arm has significantly weakened, there is a probability that eating that food may also cause you to feel "spaced out," irritable, nervous, or perceptually disturbed. Foods can be tested in sequence, with a brief pause between each test. Spit out each sample after testing.

When kinesiological testing is done by an expert, as many as fourteen muscle groups may be involved. Training for the administration of such testing is prolonged. The prime problem is the cynicism of both the public and the professions, which usually disappears when some other method is used to confirm the kinesiological findings.

My experience with many patients to whom I have demonstrated this technique has led me to usually keep a note in my pocket, to display to the patient when the test is completed and they are goggle-eyed with amazement and skepticism. The note anticipates what they will say: "I don't believe it. I think you pushed harder on my arm, the second time." Actually I have used dynamometers—instruments that scientifically measure the amount of force—and there are no such loopholes in the test.

If you try this test and find that your arm noticeably weakens on exposure to one or more foods, you can verify this startling reaction by a very simple new application of the test. Have your partner test the springiness of your arm, as he did before. Now concentrate on somebody you really dislike, and ask your partner to repeat the test. You may find that your arm again significantly weakens. The conclusions:

1. Hate destroys the vessels which contain it.
2. There is validity to kinesiological testing.

There are some physicians who utilize this method of testing, usually to corroborate results from other types of examination for allergy. In the main, however, you will find that it is chiropractors who utilize the testing. This is appropriate, since the basis for kinesiological testing was established by Dr. George Goodhart, who is himself a chiropractor.

## Intradermal Provocative Testing

The orthodox allergist performs "a scratch test," with which most readers with allergies are probably familiar. What is important is the outcome: if, by this technique, the allergist identifies pollens or other external factors to which you are allergic, he will proceed to desensitize you. Unfortunately, with food allergy this technique is not nearly as reliable and effective.

Thanks to Dr. Herbert Rinkel and Dr. Carleton Lee, a modification of the scratch test, one useful in determining food allergy, was developed. Like all new approaches in medicine, it was met with determined resistance from orthodox allergists—to the point where they conducted a lobbying campaign and succeeded in persuading the United States Food and Drug Administration to exercise its vast powers to make unavailable the liquid food concentrates that are necessary to this new method of testing. At this writing, there is a ferocious battle on between the orthodox allergists and the bioecological allergy practitioners, who do not want their patients deprived of this new and useful technique.

The usefulness of the technique lies not only in the fact that it makes diagnosis of food allergy more reliable. It also accomplishes something that orthodox allergists have never been able to do: it provides a *treatment* as well as a diagnosis of food allergy. Compare this with the outcome when you go to an orthodox allergist, are tested for food allergies, and emerge with what? A long list of foods that the allergist says you must avoid. That is the end of the line with the conventional scratch technique.

With the intradermal provocative testing, dilutions of the food, varying in concentration, are tested by injecting them intradermally (between the layers of skin). On the basis of the reactions—which usually differ widely, as the concentrations of the food differ—the physician then chooses a concentration to use by injection for treatment of the allergy. Thanks to the work of Dr. Joseph Miller, who was originally an orthodox allergist, these "neutralizing doses" were tested in double-blind experiments, which demonstrated clearly that once the appropriate dilution of the food has been identified, it *is* possible to wipe out symptoms of allergy to that food.

I write with conviction because I have personally experienced application of this principle, not in food allergy but in susceptibility to influenza. A few years ago, during an outbreak of a particularly vicious type of flu, I recognized that I had the early symptoms. As you know from your experience with this disorder, it is relentless, and medication is also palliative, rather than curative. However, I went to a bioecological allergist, who proceeded to test me with a number of dilutions of the vaccine. When he believed he had found the particular dilution that might represent a neutralizing dose, I was given an injection. Perhaps a half hour later I was free of influenza and free of the symptoms. Needless to say, if I had gone to an orthodox allergist, he would have denied the validity of such an approach and recommended aspirin for my influenza.

## Sublingual Provocative Testing

Intradermal provocative testing introduces a test substance by injection between the layers of skin; sublingual provocative testing exposes the body to the test substance by absorption from under the tongue. In this method, there is no objective way in which to appraise the patient's response—meaning that there is no wheal. The physician here relies upon subjective reports, i.e., any disturbances the patient experiences when the food has been under his tongue for a short period. This, of course, immediately alienates medicine, which is proud of its record in arriving at objective testing and avoiding reliance on subjective responses. (That hasn't quite been accomplished yet in determining what corrective lenses are needed when you have your eyes examined, but, on the other hand, it isn't apologized for, either). The orthodoxy in allergy testing therefore rejects any evaluation of this type. Yet it can be anything but a subjective response. For example, after a child was exposed to a whiff of a household germicide from a spray can, she was totally unable to draw a recognizable tree, although she had done so in great detail and with some artistic ability prior to the sublingual test. Despite evidence of this sort, though, sublingual testing is a practice largely of bioecological allergists alone.

In this test, the technician uses soluble extracts of foods, places them under the tongue, one at a time, and makes a chart of the patient's reaction. Foods are put under the tongue because absorption into the body from that area is so efficient that it is used as a means of administering nitroglycerin for patients with heart disease. In actual procedure, a few drops of a food extract are placed under the tongue and held there for about ten minutes. The examiner waits for your report on any subjective symptoms you experience, and watches you for any objective ones. One of the variables in this type of examination is the concentration of the food extract. If you have no reaction in the ten-minute period, the examiner may try a lower concentration of the same food for another ten minutes, and then a higher one. If you pass all three tests, that food is labeled as permissible for you, and the testing is resumed with another food concentrate.

It is easy to dismiss subjective reactions on the grounds that there is no way to appraise them scientifically, but some patients who are strongly allergic obviously suffer very severe allergic reponses to sublingual testing, very often to foods or drugs to which they never suspected they were sensitive. Among possible reactions are dysperception (where reality becomes twisted), or sleepiness, marked irritability, headaches, and sometimes what appear to be truly psychotic reactions. The responses during the sublingual test may or may not match those that initially brought the patient in for testing.

As with the intradermal provocative test, it is often possible to locate a neutralizing dose by using varied dilutions of the food extract. When the test administrant reaches the right dilution, the patient knows because his symptoms are relieved.

Sublingual provocative testing has some of the disadvantages of other methods. Obviously, not very many foods can be tested in a single session, and if a very pronounced reaction occurs, the accuracy of the procedure will be better maintained if the testing is temporarily discontinued, to be resumed a day or two later.

Needless to say, you should choose an allergist who has experience with this method. In Appendix I are sources for locating such a practitioner.

## Cytotoxic Testing

In cytotoxic testing, a technician observes the reaction of your white blood cells to exposure to a dried extract of a food. The list of foods to be tested always includes those that are frequent causes of allergic reactions, and is supplemented with those to which you are addicted or at least eat frequently.

When white blood cells are exposed to dried extracts of the test foods, those foods to which you are allergic will cause the cells to deteriorate. Deterioration may range from a slight effect to total destruction of the white cells, and, in part, the degree to which you are sensitive to a food is rated by the percentage of white blood cells that react adversely to the food concentrate.

This test has several advantages, one being that your only participation is supplying a sample of blood. Second, a large number of tests can be done in a relatively short period of time. Third, the count of the affected cells and the degree to which they are affected allows an evaluation of the degree of sensitivity to the test food, so that you can emerge from this test with a list of allergy foods that indicates minimal sensitivity, mild degree, moderate degree, or severe. Predicating his judgments upon this, the practitioner will tell you that some foods must be totally avoided for an indefinite period, others may be taken only at long intervals, some can be taken regularly, etc.

Unlike the intradermal provocative test, cytotoxic testing does not offer the possibility of establishing neutralizing doses, and thereby supplies no treatment, other than guiding you to avoidance or infrequent use of foods to which the white cells have proved sensitive. Second, the mechanism of the body which is involved in this reaction may not be involved in other reactions to food, and the latter will not be identified by the cytotoxic test.

My personal objections to leaning on this test too heavily are derived from my experience with many patients who have undergone this type of examination. First, the test is only as good as the technician who does it—and the capabilities of technicians do differ. Second, the test, like any other, may give false negatives. This is particularly true of foods to which you are genuinely sensitive but have not consumed for a long period of time. Third, there is little correlation between the cytotoxic test results and those derived from other methods, in part because the mechanism being evaluated in a cytotoxic test is not the same as that involved in other methods. Nonetheless, for some patients, cytotoxic testing has proved valuable, if it has done nothing more than to identify some of the causes of some of their symptoms.

## The Rast Method

Immunoglobulin E is a factor in the immune system that attempts to defend the body by attacking the antigens that are the mischief makers in hay fever and other allergic reactions. This factor not only reacts to pollen, but often interacts with specific foods consumed by the allergic individual. The Rast method measures the intensity of the reaction between the antibodies formed by the allergic individual and the antigens (foods, pollens, etc.) that initiated the reaction. What actually happens, then, in this method of testing, is a labeling of the antigen-antibody reaction by use of a radioactive substance, allowing the degree of reaction to be measured with the same type of device that is used by atomic scientists to detect radioactivity.

Like the cytotoxic and other tests, the Rast method has some disadvantages. It is applicable only to a limited number of foods, and a positive result in the test does not necessarily mean that the patient, eating the particular food, will have clinical symptoms. Moreover, this method of testing is costly.

I am aware that this instruction may be wasted on those who know that they have allergies, but it may be valuable to those who don't. The list of symptoms that can be caused by allergy would require an entire separate chapter, but among them are many the public does not link with this disorder. Consider a conversation I had with a major television personality, when we discussed his long-term battle with weight gain. Originally, he was a hypoglycemic, and, like so many sufferers with low blood sugar, he was unaware of the condition and had actually gone for treatment for "emotional" symptoms. These symptoms promptly disappeared when I suggested a glucose-tolerance test and, based on its results, his doctor placed him on a hypoglycemic diet. Subsequently, he once more gained unwanted weight, which he has a tendency to do but has fought for many years. He finally underwent a cytotoxic test, eliminated from his diet the foods to which he was sensitive, and promptly lost thirty pounds.

I tell this anecdote because it perfectly illustrates one of the hundreds of symptoms to which allergy can contribute. Yet there are very few laymen who are aware that resistant obesity can be based not on excess calories, but on eating foods to which one is allergic. This is merely an example of the multiple faces of allergy. I emphasize it because I receive so many letters from readers and radio listeners who do not realize that their hypoglycemia can lead to allergies, and that their allergies can be responsible for everything from skin rashes to constipation, from irritability to blurring of vision, from semi-psychotic behavior to learning difficulties.

## III. IDIOPATHIC POSTPRANDIAL SYNDROME

There are many patients who display the symptoms of hypoglycemia, but whose glucose-tolerance tests are judged (by the orthodox physician) to be perfectly normal. Part of the problem derives from the refusal of the orthodox to recognize that there are individual differences in reaction to changes in blood sugar levels. Another factor, which also has been discussed elsewhere in this text, resides in the methodology of the glucose-tolerance test. There is no law that says that changes in blood glucose levels must occur on the hour, and yet those are the periods in which testing is usually conducted.

There is, however, a substantial group of patients who after eating suffer an immediate drop in blood sugar levels. This is called "reactive hypoglycemia," and by proper choice of foods and management of allergies, if present, it can be controlled.

That leaves us with the last group: people who show all the symptoms of hypoglycemia—sometimes immediately after a meal, sometimes later—and whose glucose-tolerance tests are so solidly, so patently normal that the orthodoxy considers that this group literally disproves the very existence of hypoglycemia. In a recent study, published in the *Journal of the American Medical Association* and titled "Idiopathic Postprandial Syndrome," a partial explanation has been found for this phenomenon. The condition is not hypoglycemia, say the authors, but reflects an excessive activity of stimulating neurotransmitters, of adrenal origin, in the brain. Since they are unable to explain why there should be such an excessive level of adrenal hormone derivatives in the brain, they titled the syndrome "idiopathic"—which literally means that they don't know what the cause is.

They could have found the explanation in the original text of this book, published sixteen years ago. Some individuals react to a drop in blood sugar with excessive production of adrenal hormones. This can create some of the nervousness and restlessness associated with low blood sugar. It can also be responsible for the unprovoked feelings of panic and anxiety. The mechanism here is simple to understand: the body is going through an adrenal reaction, triggered by disturbances in carbohydrate metabolism, which ordinarily would be caused by tension, anxiety, or fright. There being nothing on the horizon to justify those feelings, the body reacts to its own hormone response by interpreting it as panic, anxiety, or tension. In the case of those with "idiopathic postprandial syndrome," the abnormal adrenal activity, ordinarily triggered to compensate for a drop in blood sugar, is elicited by the wrong choice of foods. The syndrome is therefore not "idiopathic." For those who have so interpreted it, let me offer a disturbing thought: despite the absence of changes in the blood sugar levels of these patients, the hypoglycemia diet nonetheless brings the symptoms under control.

# Index